ABOUT THIS BOOK

This book has been specially designed and developed to make learning easier and more productive. First, the content was determined through research and consultation with educators and practitioners. Next, topics were visually mapped out in two-page frames by a writing, illustrating, and design team. Frames were then written, illustrated, designed, and produced as a working draft. That draft was reviewed and revised through consultation with educators and practitioners and the result is the book you now have.

We believe this process produces a better text. Illustrations are never a page or two away from the text. Topics are presented completely and always in *perspective*. Information is easy to find and understand. We think you'll find it a useful guide to understanding the health care principles, career concepts, and nursing skills you need to become a home care aide.

OUR CONSULTANTS

First, we'd like to thank our Consultants for their insights, suggestions, and constructive criticism. They have helped us produce a much better book for you to use.

Laura Katz Najera, R.N., M.P.A.

Nursing Administrator
Stat Health Care Services, Inc.
Bronx, NY

Barbara Wilson, R.N., B.S.N.

Vice President, Patient Services
Lockport Memorial Hospital
Lockport, NY

Clara McElroy, R.N., M.A.

President, First Call Medical, Inc.
President, Florida Health Academy
Bonita Springs, FL

Melanie Vlosky, R.N., B.S.N., M.E.D.

Associate Director of Nursing
Amherst Nursing and Convalescent Home
Amherst, NY

Dorothy M. Witmer, Ed.D., R.N.

Supervisor of Health Occupations Education
Idaho Division of Vocational Education
Boise, ID

Dr. Peggy Sexton-Isaac

Program Area Coordinator
Department of Health Careers
Pima Community College
Pima, AZ

Paula Elberhoumi, R.N., B.S.N., M.S.

Trainer
Selfhelp Community Services
New York, NY

Though we believe this first edition is a fine book, we know that every book can always be improved. Any suggestions which you think would make the book better would be welcome. You may send them to me:

Dennis Hogan
Publisher, Perspective Press, P.O. Box 609, Tenafly, NJ 07670

HOW TO USE THIS BOOK

The two biggest differences between this book and most textbooks are the *frame-by-frame* design and the many illustrations used. Complete topics are presented on facing-pages which we call *frames*. In each frame, you can quickly see the important points in the topic. You will also see illustrations that add information and emphasis.

We suggest you:

1.) Scan the topic map for a basic understanding.

2.) Read the highlighted statements of the overview.

3.) Carefully read the complete overview.

4.) Carefully read the topic map.

5.) Repeat Steps 1-4 until you are confident that you know the material.

If you perform these steps *before* a topic is discussed in class you will learn more *during* class. Always write down in this book or a notebook any important points made by the instructor during class. That way, you won't forget them. You should then review the frame and your notes again *after* class. This will reinforce what you have learned.

TOPIC

UNIT NAME AND NUMBER

OVERVIEW

There is usually an overview at the left or top which provides you with a general explanation of the topic. Key points are highlighted.

TOPIC MAP

An illustrated map of the topic uses text and illustrations to aid understanding. The illustrations reinforce the explanation and help you to focus on important points.

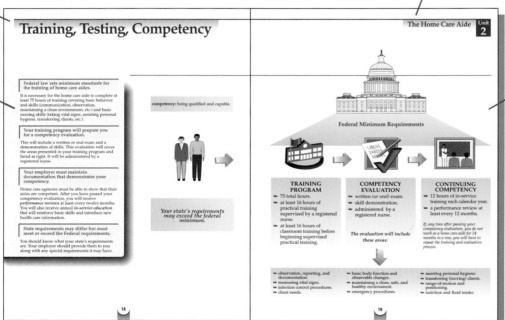

FRAME

Each pair of facing pages is a frame. It usually covers a complete topic. In a few cases, two topics are covered, and some procedures take two or more frames. You'll find a handy *Index of Frames* on the last page of the book.

LEARNING NURSING SKILLS

Most of this book covers the basic nursing skills you'll need to become a home care aide. We've standardized our frame-by-frame design for presenting these skills. This will make it easier for you to learn them by:

- Explaining the nursing principles behind the skill;
- Organizing the skill into a step-by-step procedure;
- Illustrating key points in the procedure
- Providing *Pointers* that reflect practice.

In order to develop skills, however, you must practice them. You'll do this in a supervised classroom or clinical setting where you can discuss your questions, practice procedures, and become skilled. We can't illustrate every detail of each procedure. So we've illustrated key stages. *You will only see all the details when you practice the skill.* Use this book as a guide to better understand what is important about the skill. But don't use it as a substitute for practice.

TOPIC

UNIT NAME AND NUMBER

OVERVIEW

Provides you with a general explanation of the skill. Key points are highlighted.

STEP-BY-STEP PROCEDURE

Skills are presented in natural steps. Illustrations show key stages of progress.

POINTERS

Reflect practice, offer alternatives, alert you to possible problems, etc.

TEXT BOXES

Related topics, principles, or important issues are explained.

PREPARATION AND COMPLETION SYMBOLS

We've devoted two frames to the basic principles of preparation and completion (washing hands, ensuring privacy, etc.) that you should follow every time you perform a procedure. *You should learn these principles by heart.* For reference, however, we include the page numbers for these frames. We also include the page number for the additional steps you should take for the type of procedure you are performing.

UNDERSTANDING AND LEARNING

The design of this book should make it easier for you to understand the information that is being presented. However, you also need to think about this information and ask yourself what it means to you. When something has a personal meaning to you, it is easier to understand and remember.

At the end of each unit is a *Consider* section that asks you to think about the information in the unit and consider what it means to you. You will be asked to imagine yourself or a family member as a home care client, to compare what was presented in the unit to your everyday experience, to list what seems important to you, and so on. Above all, you are being asked to think about the information and to personalize it.

Use the *Consider* sections to develop the habit of thinking about what you are learning. Then use the *Review* section to test your knowledge of the material in the unit. Write down any questions you have or topics you don't understand and ask your instructor about them in class.

UNIT NAME AND NUMBER

Personal Care

Personal Care Unit 14

CONSIDER

Think carefully about the question and answer it as well as you can. Then ask yourself if your answer tells you anything about what you've learned. Discuss your answers with your instructor.

CONSIDER

1. Describe how a bath or shower makes you feel physically. Does it affect your attitude as well? If so, how? What about a clean change of clothing?

2. Beginning with the start of the day, list as many of your personal care habits as you can: how and when you like to bathe, shampoo, brush your teeth, change clothes, etc. Are there any habits that it would bother you to change? Which ones? Why?

3. In what ways do you notice the personal hygiene and grooming of others? How does this influence your opinion of them?

4. If you needed someone to perform your personal care, what guidelines would you give them? How would you like them to treat you?

REVIEW

Key Terms – Test your understanding of each of these first. Then use each one once to fill in the incomplete statements below.

universal precautions
flossing
oral care
dentures
bed bath
105-110 degrees
perineal care
tub bath or shower
shampooing
massaging

1. Clients who must stay in bed are given a _____, in which the client's entire body is washed a part at a time.

2. After _____, you will brush the client's hair as they like it.

3. _____ is provided every two hours to unconscious clients to keep them from aspirating saliva.

4. You must practice _____ when providing oral hygiene or shaving a client because of the possibility of coming in contact with the client's blood.

5. When assisting a client taking a _____ you must be alert to safety hazards such as slippery surfaces, overly hot water, or temporary dizziness.

6. _____ the skin relaxes the client and stimulates circulation, which helps to prevent the development of decubitus ulcers.

7. _____ are false teeth that are form-fitted to the gums and must be cleaned as often as natural teeth.

8. _____ is a safe temperature range for bathing water.

9. _____ teeth removes tartar and food particles from surfaces difficult to clean with a toothbrush.

10. _____ involves cleaning the genitals, anus, and the area between (the *perineum*).

210

211

REVIEW

Review your understanding of the key terms first. Then test your knowledge by using them to complete the statements. You can find the answers in the unit if you have difficulty.

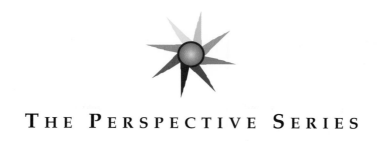

THE PERSPECTIVE SERIES

Home Care Aide

for Hannah

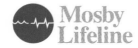
Mosby
Lifeline

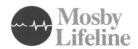

Publisher: David Culverwell
Managing Editor: Doris Smith
Assistant Editor: Jennifer Roe

First Edition
Copyright © 1995 by Mosby-Year Book, Inc.
A Mosby Lifeline imprint of Mosby-Year Book, Inc.

Printed in the United States of America.

Mosby-Year Book, Inc.
11830 Westline Industrial Drive
St. Louis, Missouri 63146

International Standard Book Number
0-8151-4748-1

95 96 97 98 99 / 9 8 7 6 5 4 3 2 1

Home Care Aide

TABLE OF CONTENTS

FOUNDATIONS

Home Care Aide
TABLE OF CONTENTS

NURSING CARE

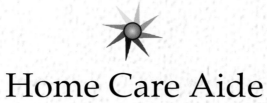

Home Care Aide

TABLE OF CONTENTS

ACKNOWLEDGEMENTS

All of our consultants were invaluable but two of them also contributed material to this book. I'd like to give them special thanks for their contributions:

Laura Najera   Stat Health Care

Barbara Wilson   Lockport Memorial Hospital

In addition to our consultants, there are a number of very talented people I'd like to thank: Richard Maran (the conceptual wizard of maranGraphics), Rob Maran (maranGraphics' technical specialist), and all the people at maranGraphics who helped with this book; Peter Baranowski of OKOM Design who designed it; Tamara Newnam, our lead artist, who drew most of the art and did a great job; Dave Culverwell and Doris Smith of Mosby Lifeline for their support and assistance; Chris Baumle and Dave Orzechowski of Mosby for their production help; Melanie Wilson for her insights; Denny Curtin for his advice and example; and above all, Joan, Joan, and Hannah for their support, assistance, and encouragement.

Dennis Hogan, *Publisher*

Perspective Press

NOTICE

FOREWORD

Throughout this book, we have tried to emphasize the importance of the client in home care. However, we'd like to take this opportunity before you begin your training to say it again. We think it is impossible to over-emphasize the importance of the client. Being sensitive to the client's feelings, concerns, problems, desires, beliefs, habits, and everything else that makes each client an individual is as necessary for home care aides as knowing the skills.

In using this book and taking your training, it will be natural to focus on the information and skills required to be a home care aide. There is a lot to learn. Always try to remember, however, that the most important thing about being a home care aide is that you are helping people.

We've tried to point out the concerns and rights that clients have wherever we can. We've also asked questions in the *Consider* sections at the end of each unit that should help you to think about clients as people. Imagining yourself, your family, and your friends as home care clients should remind you how special and important each person is and help you treat each client the way you would like to be treated.

Health Care

Health care in America is constantly changing.

One hundred years ago, health care for most Americans was seen as the physician who treated all illnesses and conditions. Only patients with the most serious illnesses and disorders went to a hospital, and many of these patients died. The hospital as a medical center where the sick could get well was a new idea.

Since that time, there has been a rapid growth in the type and amount of health care available.

Today, we have a large system of highly specialized health care services and care givers in many settings. Home care is a very important part of this system. *Home care aides,* working for *home care agencies,* provide basic nursing care and other services to people living at home. In many cases, these people would otherwise have to be institutionalized in a hospital or nursing home.

What makes health care succeed is teamwork.

As a home care aide, you will be an important part of a *home care team,* working with medical, nursing, and service personnel to provide health care. You will need to learn about the members of this team, their roles, and your own in order to perform your duties. You will also need to learn about clients' rights and needs and what you must do to provide for them.

Primary locations of professional health care:

Physician's Office

The physician's office is where most people go for *primary care*: care for the many day-to-day health problems that do not require hospitalization or specialized medical care. They receive check-ups, general health care, diagnosis and treatment of minor illnesses, and advice on getting specialized care when it is needed.

Hospitals

Hospitals provide specialized care for the treatment of serious illness. The type of service depends on the size and nature of the hospital, with major medical centers and teaching hospitals (where medical students are trained) offering the most services.

Home

Home care is generally much less expensive than institutional care and has many social and psychological advantages for the people receiving it. It is often provided by *home care aides* working for a *home care agency.* All types of people receive home care: young, old, disabled, people recovering from surgery or illness, etc. Home care may be provided for short or long periods. The people who receive it are called the home care agency's *clients.* In some cases, two home care agencies may be involved in a client's care: one managing the client's case and one providing the actual service.

Long-Term Care Facility

These facilities are also known as *nursing homes* because of the nursing care they provide. People receiving care live in the facility and are called *residents.* Most residents are elderly. Much of the care they receive is performed by nursing assistants working under the supervision of a registered nurse (RN).

Hospices

Hospices provide care for the dying and their families. They try to make the dying patient as comfortable as possible. They include the family in their program so that the patient will not feel alone. Hospice care can be provided in the home, in a hospice facility, and in many long-term care facilities.

Home Care

The goal of home care is to meet clients' medical, nursing, psychological, and social needs in the home.

There are many advantages to home care over institutional care: familiar surroundings, greater feeling of independence, nearness of family and friends, lower cost, etc. However, these advantages may not matter if the home care aide fails to provide good care. Your job, and your agency's, is to provide care that helps the client to enjoy as good a quality of life as possible.

Home care agencies provide environmental services, personal care, and health care.

Many people with disorders or disabilities need help in maintaining their *home environment:* making beds, cleaning rooms, doing laundry, etc. They often need someone to prepare meals or to help with personal care (bathing, dressing, using the toilet, etc.). They may also need health care.

Much of this care is performed by home care aides.

Different amounts of training are required to perform these services, with health care requiring the most. The type of health care provided by home care aides is basic nursing care. Home care agencies have a *registered nurse (R.N.)* who supervises the licensed nurses and home care aides on staff. The nursing staff works with other health care professionals as a *home care team* providing care for the client.

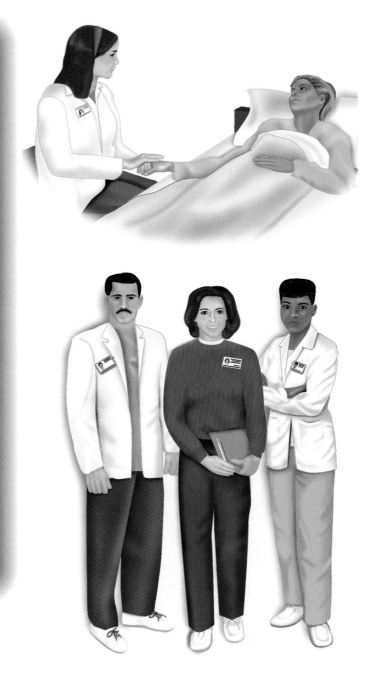

> **environment:** surrounding conditions, influences, or circumstances.

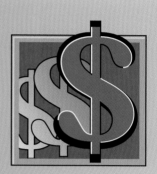

Paying for Home Care

Home care is generally much less expensive than care in a hospital or nursing home, but it is still costly. While some clients may pay for it through insurance or their own resources, many rely on federal and state payments. Medicare is a federal program for people 65 or older, though it also covers people under 65 with certain disabilities. Medicaid is a joint federal and state program for low-income patients. Both programs are widely used to pay for home care.

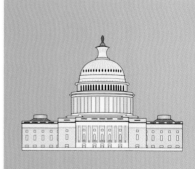

Regulation

There are federal laws regarding clients' rights, the training and supervision of home care aides, and the operation of home care agencies. The goal of these laws is to ensure quality client care by a trained staff. Many states have additional regulations for home care agencies and regularly evaluate whether agencies meet these requirements. Home care agencies must meet federal and state requirements to receive Medicare and Medicaid payments for their services.

The Home Care Team

The *home care team* is made up of specialized teams working with the client.

Together, they prepare and maintain a *care plan* that meets a client's medical, nursing, psychological, and social needs in the client's home.

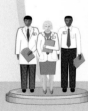

THE MEDICAL TEAM

All clients have an **attending physician** responsible for the medical aspects of their care plan. Depending on their condition, clients may also have one or more physician specialists, including a psychiatrist, attending to their care. Each client's care plan must be reviewed regularly by his or her attending physician.

THE NURSING TEAM

Home care aides are part of the nursing team. A **registered nurse (RN),** often with special training in **Public Health Nursing,** supervises the nursing team and regularly evaluates the client's care plan. **Licensed practical nurses (LPN)** provide nursing services and assist the RN. The home care agency's nursing staff will be supervised by an RN who is called **Director of Nursing** (or Home Care, Patient Services, etc.). Depending on the agency, one of the responsibilities of the nursing staff can be to train new home care aides.

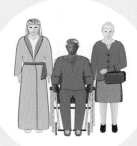

THE CLIENT

The client is the central member of the health care team. Clients can assist in their own care through cooperation and taking an active role. In addition, the client's family plays an important role and needs to be considered along with the client.

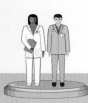

THE SERVICE TEAM

In addition to the nursing and medical teams, there are many other health care specialists who may work on the client's health care team. These include: ▼ A **social worker** to provide the social services that clients can't provide themselves. ▼ A **physical therapist** or an **occupational therapist** to help injured or disabled clients regain lost physical functions. ▼ A **dietician** to plan the diet.

Clients' Rights

All citizens have rights which protect them.

These rights include all the rights guaranteed by government, such as freedom from discrimination, freedom of religion, property rights, etc. In addition, home care clients also have many medical and human rights specific to health care.

Federal and state laws guarantee special rights for clients of home care agencies.

These laws protect the client's right to quality health care and good treatment. They include rights regarding client participation, quality of care, costs of care, training of home care aides, and services provided.

Clients must be fully informed of their rights.

Clients must be informed of their rights and all regulations and rules that will affect them **in writing before care is provided.** This written *bill of rights* must be in language that the client can understand. In many states, clients have to sign this as proof that they have been informed. Though federal regulations are the same for all states, state regulations differ. You must know your state's regulations regarding clients' rights.

Rights of Clients

These rights pay special attention to the home care client's right to quality care by trained personnel. Home care aides must respect and honor these rights.

Clients must be free to exercise these rights without interference, pressure, discrimination, punishment, or any other actions that make exercising their rights difficult.

The client's family or guardian may exercise these rights if the client has been judged incompetent.

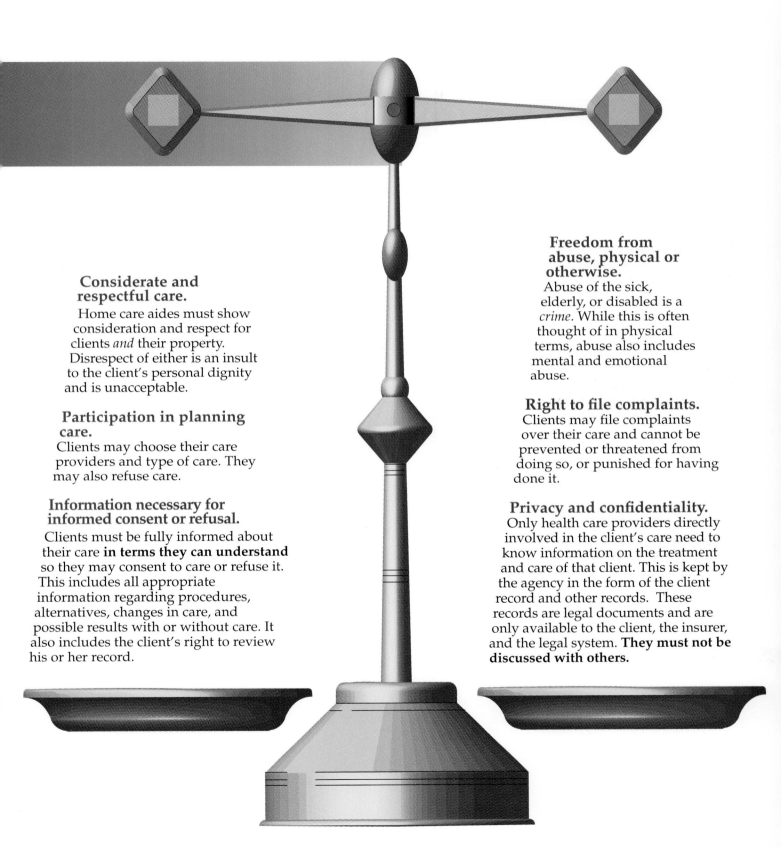

Considerate and respectful care.

Home care aides must show consideration and respect for clients *and* their property. Disrespect of either is an insult to the client's personal dignity and is unacceptable.

Participation in planning care.

Clients may choose their care providers and type of care. They may also refuse care.

Information necessary for informed consent or refusal.

Clients must be fully informed about their care **in terms they can understand** so they may consent to care or refuse it. This includes all appropriate information regarding procedures, alternatives, changes in care, and possible results with or without care. It also includes the client's right to review his or her record.

Freedom from abuse, physical or otherwise.

Abuse of the sick, elderly, or disabled is a *crime*. While this is often thought of in physical terms, abuse also includes mental and emotional abuse.

Right to file complaints.

Clients may file complaints over their care and cannot be prevented or threatened from doing so, or punished for having done it.

Privacy and confidentiality.

Only health care providers directly involved in the client's care need to know information on the treatment and care of that client. This is kept by the agency in the form of the client record and other records. These records are legal documents and are only available to the client, the insurer, and the legal system. **They must not be discussed with others.**

Home Care

1.
Think of examples of teamwork in which you have participated (e.g., at work, in sports, in civic activities, etc.). What makes a team successful?

2.
Imagine that you are a person who needs home care. How would you want your home care team to work with you? With each other?

3.
If you were a person needing home care, what concerns would you have about your quality of life?

4.
If you were a home care client, which rights do you think would mean the most to you? Why?

REVIEW

clients

Medicare and Medicaid

home care team

care plan

registered nurse

clients' rights

personal dignity

informed consent

privacy and confidentiality

1. A _____ supervises the duties and work of the home care aide.

2. Being given all necessary information about their care in terms they can understand is necessary for clients to give _____.

3. People receiving home care from a home care agency are called _____.

4. The right to _____ means that only health care providers directly involved in the client's care may share information about that client's care.

5. Federal and state laws guarantee _____.

6. Home care agencies must meet federal and state standards to be able to receive _____ payments.

7. Each client's _____ is developed by the registered nurse and reviewed by the physician responsible for the client's care.

8. The client is the central member of the _____ , which also includes medical, nursing, and service personnel.

9. Health care must be considerate and respectful of the client's _____ .

The Home Care Aide

Home care aides perform a major role in home care.

Home care aides increase the ability of nurses and physicians to provide care. They are an important part of the home care team and necessary to the operation of home care agencies.

The home care aide must follow the regulations that apply to his or her job.

Federal, state, and professional requirements regulate training, competency, practices, and behavior. They are a *legal* definition of how to become, be, and stay a home care aide. You must obey these regulations because, as a home care aide, you will be entering into a legal relationship with the client and your employer.

There are also personal requirements necessary to be a home care aide.

You will be working with people, providing a personal service. The standards for this are as high as the standards by which you treat yourself and by which you like to be treated. Consider, too, that the people you serve have had their lives affected by age, illness, or disability. You must pay special attention to how you treat them. Your attitude, behavior, and appearance are all a part of that.

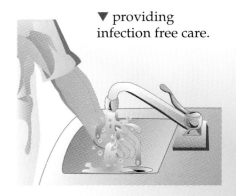

▼ providing infection free care.

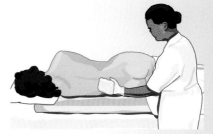

▼ assisting with personal care.

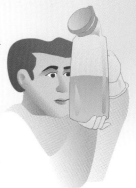

▼ assisting with elimination.

NEVER perform any activity that is not specifically part of your training, certification, and job description even if you think you understand how to do it, or are requested to do it by anyone, including your supervisor.

NEVER try any activity you do not understand. Ask your supervisor to explain it so you understand it.

▼ moving and positioning clients.

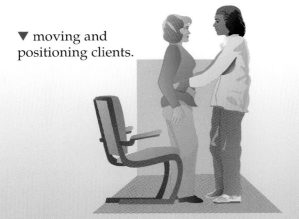

▼ bedmaking and housekeeping.

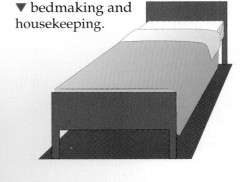

The Job of the Home Care Aide

The home care aide works under a registered nurse's supervision and assists the nurse in providing basic nursing care to clients. Your employer (in a detailed *job description*) and your nursing supervisor will tell you specifically which nursing care activities you will perform. You should also ask your supervisor or employer for a copy of all regulations affecting your duties and you should memorize them.

▼ preparing and serving food and fluids.

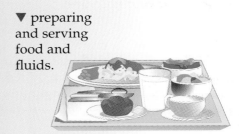

▼ measuring vital signs.

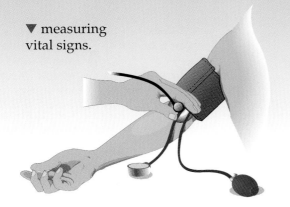

▼ preventive and restorative care.

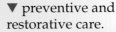

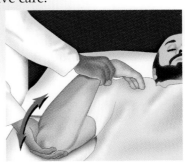

Personal Characteristics

Attitude matters.

Your attitude will affect the clients and other members of the home care team with whom you will work. If you consider how much more you enjoy being with people who are enthusiastic, friendly, and cheerful, you can see how much more effective you will be if you have a good attitude.

Ethical behavior is necessary.

Ethics are standards of conduct based on morals. Your behavior must show the characteristics outlined on these pages for you to succeed as a home care aide. Consider these to be personal requirements for the job.

You must be responsible and dependable.

The client and your agency will depend upon your performing your job in the client's home without direct on-site supervision. You must show up when you are expected and do what you required to do.

Understanding yourself is a key to helping others.

Think about the personal requirements for the job and honestly consider any areas in which you need to improve. Try to see yourself as others see you. How clients and co-workers see you will influence your effectiveness and that of the home care team.

There are legal aspects to many of these personal requirements.

Failing to practice them will hurt your job performance and can violate your clients' rights. Practicing them will increase your success and enjoyment as a home care aide.

HONESTY AND TRUSTWORTHINESS

You will be trusted in the client's home without on-site supervision. You must perform the duties that are asked of you and report exactly what you have done or observed to your supervisor.

CONSIDERATION AND PATIENCE

Each client is unique. Your interaction with clients will be more successful if you recognize that some may need more time, assistance, or encouragement to perform activities than others.

CONFIDENTIALITY
You must not discuss information about the client or the client's treatment with anyone not directly involved in the treatment of the client.

DEDICATION AND DEPENDABILITY
You must always do everything that is expected of you, when and how it is expected, even though no one may be watching.

PRACTICE THE GOLDEN RULE

Treat others as you wish them to treat you.

COOPERATION AND COMMUNICATION
You are a member of a team that relies on your performance.
As a home care aide, you will often have the closest view of the client. Your observations about the client's condition will be critical to the client's care.

COURTESY AND RESPECT
This will improve all your relations with clients and co-workers.

Health, Hygiene, & Appearance

You must maintain good physical and mental health.

Your job requires thinking, understanding, coordination, and strength that can be hurt by poor health habits. You need good health habits that will keep you rested and alert and keep you from becoming physically or mentally run-down.

Your must have good personal hygiene.

You will work closely with clients. Bad breath or body odor (including strong deodorants and perfumes) will hurt your ability to perform your duties. An unclean body or clothes will also offend clients and may violate requirements for infection free care.

You must present a professional appearance.

Your uniform and personal clothing must be neat, clean, and functional. Shoes should be comfortable. Clothes should fit to allow the freedom of movement necessary to perform your duties. Hair should be well-groomed and pulled back if long. Fingernails should be neat and trim. Don't wear jewelry or heavy make-up.

HEALTH

- ✔ has a nutritious, well-balanced, diet.
- ✔ exercises regularly and is physically fit.
- ✔ gets enough sleep to be well-rested.
- ✔ finds ways to relax and reduce stress.
- ✔ avoids drugs, except as prescribed by a doctor.
- ✔ doesn't use alcohol on the job or abuse it off the job.

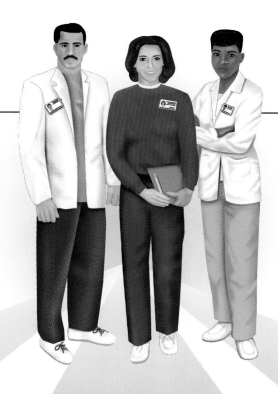

HYGIENE

✔ bathes or showers daily.
✔ cleans hands regularly.
✔ keeps teeth clean and breath fresh.
✔ has no noticeable body odor or fragrances.

APPEARANCE

✔ wears required clothing and identification.
✔ wears clothes that fit comfortably and neatly.
✔ wears shoes that fit correctly and comfortably.
✔ keeps clothing clean.
✔ keeps hair clean, neat, and off the shoulder.
✔ doesn't wear jewelry that can scratch or be pulled.
✔ doesn't wear heavy make-up.

Your employer will have requirements for your health, hygiene, and appearance. Learn these requirements and practice habits that help you to meet them on a regular basis.

Training, Testing, Competency

Federal law sets minimum standards for the training of home care aides.

It is necessary for the home care aide to complete at least 75 hours of training covering basic behavior and skills (communication, observation, maintaining a clean environment, etc.) and basic nursing skills (taking vital signs, assisting personal hygiene, transferring clients, etc.).

Your training program will prepare you for a competency evaluation.

This will include a written or oral exam and a demonstration of skills. This evaluation will cover the areas presented in your training program and listed at right. It will be administered by a registered nurse.

Your employer must maintain documentation that demonstrates your competency.

Home care agencies must be able to show that their aides are competent. After you have passed your competency evaluation, you will receive *performance reviews* at least every twelve months. You will also receive annual *in-service education* that will reinforce basic skills and introduce new health care information.

State requirements may differ but must meet or exceed the Federal requirements.

You should know what your state's requirements are. Your employer should provide them to you along with any special requirements it may have.

competency: being qualified and capable.

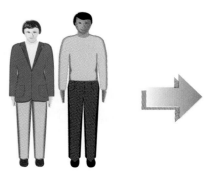

Your state's requirements may exceed the federal minimum.

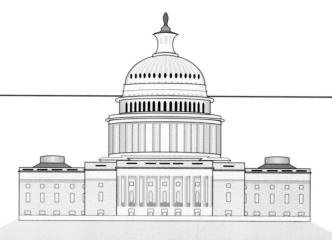

Federal Minimum Requirements

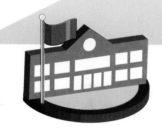 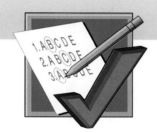 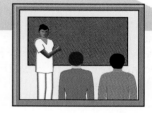

TRAINING PROGRAM

➡ 75 total hours.
➡ at least 16 hours of practical training supervised by a registered nurse.
➡ at least 16 hours of classroom training before beginning supervised practical training.

COMPETENCY EVALUATION

➡ written (or oral) exam.
➡ skill demonstration.
➡ administered by a registered nurse.

The evaluation will include these areas:

CONTINUING COMPETENCY

➡ 12 hours of in-service training each calendar year.
➡ a performance review at least every 12 months.

If, any time after passing your competency evaluation, you do not work as a home care aide for 24 months in a row, you will have to repeat the training and evaluation process.

➡ observation, reporting, and documentation.
➡ measuring vital signs.
➡ infection control procedures.
➡ client needs.

➡ basic body function and observable changes.
➡ maintaining a clean, safe, and healthy environment.
➡ emergency procedures.

➡ assisting personal hygiene.
➡ transferring (moving) clients.
➡ range-of-motion and positioning.
➡ nutrition and fluid intake.

Legal Issues

There are federal and state laws that regulate your actions as a home care aide.

These are in addition to the basic criminal and civil laws of society. This means that crimes like assault, theft, discrimination, etc., are punishable just as they would be outside your job. It also means that there are laws covering negligence, physical and mental abuse, privacy, and so on that are specific to your work.

Clients' rights are important legal requirements for the actions of home care aides.

If a client does not understand and agree to an action, you may not be allowed to perform it. Your agency will give you a complete copy of the client's rights. You should memorize them, because if you violate any of these rights, you are breaking a law.

You must report your job activity truthfully.

Client care depends upon complete and correct information. Failing to provide it may hurt the client's care and result in legal action against you. You must report any instances of misconduct by yourself or others.

You are legally responsible for your conduct.

This is called *liability.* It means that you can be prosecuted for any instance of legal misconduct, even if you were directed to do it by a supervisor or client. Conviction could result in your suspension, fines, or imprisonment.

Your training prepares you and the law requires you to act professionally. If you do not, you may be prosecuted.

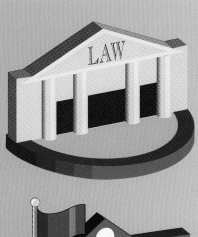

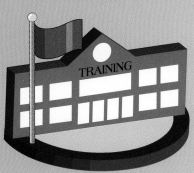

PROFESSIONAL CONDUCT

✔ Respects clients rights.

✔ Behaves ethically.

✔ Performs job as required.

✔ Follows rules and regulations of agency.

✔ Does not do anything for which he or she is not trained.

MISCONDUCT

✖ *Breaking confidentiality* requirements.

✖ *Negligence*, in failing to provide appropriate care.

✖ *Physical or mental abuse*, or poor care.

✖ *Battery*—any unauthorized touching of another person.

✖ *Theft or destruction of property.*

✖ *False imprisonment*—any unauthorized restraint of another person.

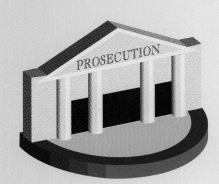

The Home Care Aide

1.

Ethical behavior (confidentiality, honesty, dependability, etc.) is a requirement for home care aides. Make a list of the benefits of such behavior from the view of your clients and employer.

2.

List ways in which poor physical or mental health could interfere with your ability to perform your duties. Do the same for poor hygiene and appearance.

3.

Consider how you can get the most out of your training. What do you think are good study habits, good classroom habits? Can you think of ways to practice your skills?

4.

Imagine that a co-worker neglects a client's care or reports false information. What are the ways this might affect the client and that client's care?

REVIEW

ethical behavior

physical and mental fitness

personal hygiene

professional appearance

federal requirements

competency evaluation

in-service training

performance review

liability

1. Home care aides must receive a _____ that evaluates their continuing competency at least every 12 months.

2. Your _____ for your actions as a home care aide means you can be prosecuted for misconduct in the performance of your job.

3. Home care aides must maintain _____ that is clean, healthy, and free of bad breath and body odor.

4. Honesty, confidentiality, and dependability are characteristics of _____ , and a personal requirement for home care aides.

5. A_____ requires good grooming and clothing that is clean, neat, comfortable, and functional.

6. Home care aide training programs must meet _____ _____ for at least 75 hours of training in specific content areas.

7. The _____ for home care aides includes a written exam and a demonstration of skills.

8. Proper nutrition, regular exercise, recreation, and rest are necessary for_____.

9. Home care agencies must provide aides with a minimum of 12 hours of _____ each calendar year.

Communication

You have not communicated unless you have been understood.

Communication is the exchange of information between people. Your job requires you to communicate regularly with clients and co-workers. Because the health and welfare of clients is at stake, you must be clear, accurate, and understandable.

You are constantly communicating even when you are not speaking or writing.

Communication can be through words *(verbal)*, acts *(nonverbal)*, or both. Nonverbal communication does not have to be active. Your clothing, body language, facial expressions, and general appearance communicate information *at all times.* They should be in keeping with the personal and professional requirements already discussed.

Empathy, your ability to understand things from another person's view, is necessary for good communication.

Careful listening and observation are required. This is especially true wherever there are cultural, physical, religious, or other basic differences between people.

Knowing your role and its requirements is also necessary for good communication.

This provides you with the basis to understand others and to make yourself understood. Your employer will have specific requirements for reporting client information and for other communications with clients and co-workers.

Developing good communication skills takes effort and practice. It will increase your effectiveness and success and will keep you from communicating wrong information.

24

LISTENING:

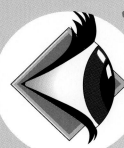

✔ Don't assume you know what is being communicated or you may miss the point.

✔ Show interest in what you are hearing.

✔ Be patient. Let others tell you information in their own words.

✔ Ask questions about anything you do not understand.

✔ Repeat back your understanding of what was said.

OBSERVING:

✔ Be alert to conditions (physical, mental, cultural, etc.) that will affect communication.

✔ Be alert to changes in condition or habit.

✔ Respect clients' and co-workers' privacy.

SPEAKING:

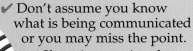
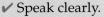
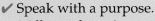
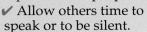

✔ Speak clearly.

✔ Speak with a purpose.

✔ Allow others time to speak or to be silent.

✔ Keep opinions to yourself.

WRITING:

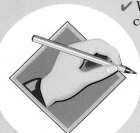

✔ Write so that your meaning cannot be mistaken. The client's health will depend on it.

✔ Be concise.

✔ Write clearly.

✔ Use ink.

NONVERBAL ACTION:

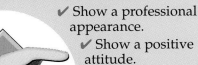
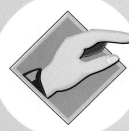

✔ Show a professional appearance.

✔ Show a positive attitude.

✔ Keep physical contact with clients gentle and respectful.

Documentation

The Client's Record

Home care agencies use a number of documents to record each client's treatment both as a way for the home care team to communicate and as a permanent legal record.

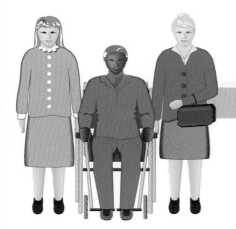

Admission

The Care Plan

ADMISSION

The attending physician refers the client to a home care agency. Clients are accepted for care if their medical, nursing, psychological, and social needs can be met by the agency in the client's home.

INITIAL EVALUATION

An evaluation performed by the registered nurse responsible for the client's case to confirm the client's condition. It becomes a baseline tool for completion of the care plan.

THE CARE PLAN

A plan of care is developed to address the client's medical, nursing, psychological, and social needs. It includes:

- types of services;
- equipment;
- rehabilitation potential;
- frequency of visits;
- activities permitted;
- nutritional requirements;
- medications and treatments;
- safety measures.

The registered nurse responsible for the client's care regularly evaluates whether the care plan meets the client's needs and will discuss changes to the plan with the client's physician, social worker, and other appropriate members of the home care team.

Home care aides are the eyes and ears of the home care team. They help in the maintenance and revision of the care plan by observing clients and reporting their observations to their nursing supervisor. Reporting requirements differ by agency. Know what types of information your supervisor needs from you and what forms you are required to use.

NOTE:
The client's record is sometimes called "the client's chart" and recording this information is often called "charting." Terminology and the number of forms differ by agency.

Aide Care

ACTIVITY SHEET

A form listing the activities to be performed by the client and/or home care aide. These activities are directly based on the care plan for the client. Activities may be performed by the client (*self*) or *assisted* by the aide. Home care agencies may ask their aides to check (✔) activities performed and sign the sheet. Clients may also be asked to sign the sheet.

I&O SHEET

A form for recording fluid intake and output. Many clients have medical conditions that require the home care aide to monitor and record this information.

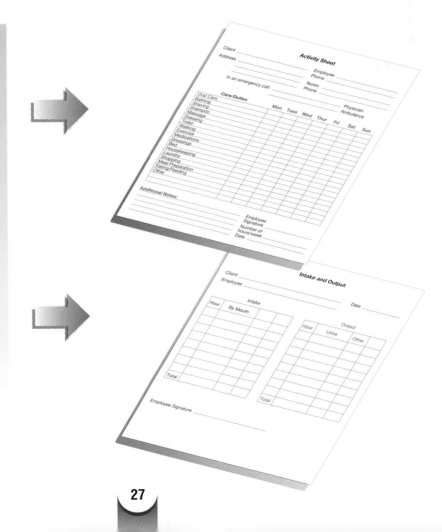

Observing & Reporting Information

Reporting client information is a primary responsibility of your job.

Besides affecting the treatment of the client, the quality of your reports will reflect directly on you and will be an important consideration in your annual performance review.

The quality of your observation skills will determine the quality of the information you gather.

What you see, hear, feel, and smell on the job is important to the client's care. The client and your co-workers depend upon your correctly reporting information from your work with the client.

You must learn the difference between *subjective* and *objective information.*

Subjective information includes things you are told or guess at. (For example, if clients tell you they are not feeling well.) *Objective information* includes things you see, hear, feel, smell, or measure. (For example, if you see redness or swelling on an area of the client's skin.) You will be asked to report both types of information and must be able to tell the difference.

Agency regulations will tell you what and how you need to report.

Learn the kind of information you will be expected to report and how you are to report it.

INFORMATION

- ◆ Measurements of temperature, pulse, respiration, blood pressure, solid and liquid intake, urine output, and weight.
- ◆ Client activities (self or assisted) such as bathing, bedrest, ambulation, sleep, and movement.

CLIENT'S RECORD

The client's record is confidential - don't discuss information about clients outside of the client's home care team!

◆ Physical conditions such as edema (swelling), color, skin irritation, body odors, breathing difficulty, abdominal firmness, gas, coughing, and wound drainage.

◆ Mental conditions such as awareness, orientation, hyperactivity, and consciousness.

◆ Client statements about pain or discomfort, appetite and diet, or other concerns.

◆ Emergency conditions like falls, fires, and rapid changes in client condition.

REPORTING PRACTICE

The client's record is a legal document.

✔ Write legibly with ink and always use an understandable signature.

✔ Draw lines through mistakes and initial them. Don't white-out or erase mistakes.

✔ Draw lines through unused spaces so they cannot be filled in later.

The client's record is a central tool of treatment.

✔ Reports must be factual and exact.

✔ You must distinguish between what you observe and what clients tell you—use quotes for clients' comments.

✔ Use the medical terminology indicated by your agency.

✔ Pay careful attention to the time of actions.

✔ Be brief and to the point

Communication

1.

Think of the last time something you said was misunderstood by someone. Why did it happen? What could *you* have said or done that would have communicated your idea better?

2.

Think of the last time you misunderstood someone else. What could *you* have done to make sure you understood what you were told? Make a list of your listening and speaking habits that you could improve.

3.

Make a list of all the things you can observe about people when you are with them. Think of a few different situations (work, family, recreation, etc.) in which to do this.

4.

Think of the last time you had trouble reading someone else's writing or someone had trouble reading yours. What can you do to make sure your handwriting is always readable?

REVIEW

**Key Terms – Test your understanding of each of these first.
Then use each one once to fill in the incomplete statements below.**

verbal communication

nonverbal communication

empathy

client's record

initial evaluation

care plan

activity sheet

I&O sheet

objective information

subjective information

1. The _____ is the collection of documents used by home care agencies to record each client's condition and treatment.

2. _____ includes things you are told or guess at.

3. The _____ for each client, based directly on the care plan, lists activities to be performed by the client and/or aide.

4. _____, such as body language and actions, is a way you communicate in addition to _____ (speaking and writing).

5. A registered nurse performs an _____ on a client which will be a baseline tool for the care plan.

6. _____ includes things you can see, hear, feel, smell, or measure.

7. Your ability to understand things from another person's view is called _____.

8. The _____ records fluid intake and output.

9. The _____ addresses the client's medical, nursing, psychological, and social needs.

Basic Client Needs

The client is a person, not an illness or condition.

Honoring each person as an individual is a guiding principle of health care and meets a basic human need.

All people have the same kinds of basic needs.

A useful way to look at this is the hierarchy of five basic needs described by the psychologist Abraham Maslow: physiological (the lowest level), safety, love and belongingness, esteem, and self-actualization (the highest level). People generally have to satisfy one level of need before they can satisfy the next level. The goal is self-fulfillment.

The home care aide helps clients satisfy as many of their basic needs as possible.

A fundamental step in this process is assisting the client to provide as much self-care as possible for the *activities of daily living* such as eating, bathing, dressing, etc. The more self-care clients can provide, the greater their sense of independence and self-esteem.

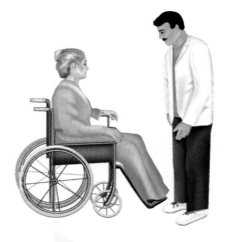

The home care aide helps each client to satisfy his or her needs. Maslow's Hierarchy at right describes the basic needs of every person.

hierarchy: A group or system of things ranked in order.

Needs

Failure to satisfy needs will cause frustration, anger, helplessness, depression, etc.

Self–Actualization
Achieving what you are capable of achieving.

Esteem
The esteem of others and oneself (which leads to the esteem of others).

Belongingness & Love
Support and affection from relationships and roles with family, friends, and society.

Safety
Security for person and property (including money).

Physiological
Eating, drinking, elimination, sexual contact, shelter, etc.

Illness & Disability

Illnesses and disabilities can make satisfying the most basic needs more difficult.

An illness is a loss of *health*. A disability is a loss of *function*. Serious illnesses, mental disorders, and physical disabilities require special care and consideration. In such cases, the home care agency must provide for *both* the client's basic needs *and* special needs.

Illness and physical disability often have a serious psychological impact.

It is normal for an illness or physical disability to cause feelings of dependence and inadequacy, which in turn can lead to depression, frustration, or resentment. Clients may express these feelings to you directly or they may do so indirectly by not cooperating in their care.

Cognitive impairment presents special difficulties for care.

Cognitively impaired clients may have difficulty understanding others. They may also have difficulty in performing normal tasks. This can be frustrating and irritating to them and can sometimes result in dangerous situations of which they may not be aware. It is important to understand the type of impairment for such clients and how best to communicate with them. It is also important to understand that they deserve respect and consideration.

depression: sadness, discouragement, gloominess.

cognitive: ability to think, know, or understand.

impairment: a weakening or reduction.

The home care aide must accept and respect the ill or disabled client's feelings and be sensitive to the special needs of such clients.

PHYSICAL DISABILITY

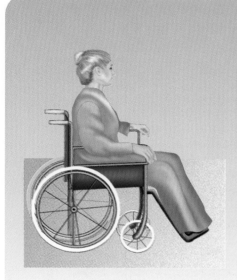

Physical disabilities such as paralysis, loss of limbs, and eyesight and hearing disorders can cause powerful feelings of frustration and helplessness. With the right assistive devices, *prostheses* (artificial body parts), and assistance, disabled clients may be able to perform self-care that would otherwise be impossible. This will increase their independence, improve their quality of life, and help them to feel good about themselves.

The goal of the home care aide is to help clients with disabilities achieve as much self-care as possible. Hearing aids, special eating utensils, walkers, wheelchairs, and prostheses are among the items that are used by disabled clients to provide self-care. When working with physically disabled clients, home care aides should be:

- sensitive to the clients' feelings;
- respectful of their mental *and* physical abilities;
- familiar with the assistive items they use (see pages 274-275);
- encouraging and positive about their efforts at self-care.

COGNITIVE IMPAIRMENT

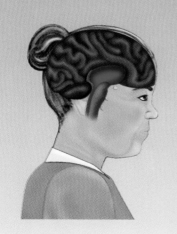

The brain of cognitively impaired people does not allow them to understand, remember, or think in normal ways. People can be born cognitively impaired or can develop it in later life from physiological causes. *Mental retardation* and *autism* are types of cognitive impairment people have at birth. Strokes, brain injuries, Alzheimer's disease, illness, and medication are among the physiological causes of cognitive impairment developed after birth.

Physiologically caused cognitive impairment that gets worse and worse, until all cognitive ability is lost, is called *dementia. Alzheimer's disease* is the most common cause of dementia. An early symptom is forgetfulness which progresses to complete loss of emotional and intellectual control and then death. These clients often become more confused or agitated late in the day, a condition known as *sundowning*.

Communication with the cognitively impaired is difficult but can be performed with:

- a gentle touch;
- simple and direct instructions;
- a comforting and patient manner.

Family, Customs, Values

The client's home is a place of *family, customs, and values.* In addition to their health, each person's life is built upon family relationships, religious beliefs, and cultural heritage. In many cases, these aspects of their lives will influence their care. The family is especially important in home care. Whether the family is in the home or outside it, it plays an important part in satisfying the client's needs and in the success of the client's care.

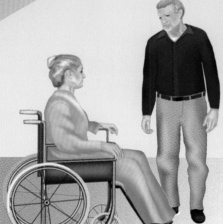

FAMILY

Family relationships are often the most meaningful parts of a person's life. They can be a source of pleasure and strength, but also of pain and stress. Whatever the nature of the relationship, the client's feelings about it are often intense.

The relationships of clients and their families are complex. The family may be psychologically or financially dependent upon the client, or the reverse may be true. The family may or may not be supportive of the client. There may be many conflicts between family members.

The client's family frequently plays a major role in the client's care by creating a positive or negative environment for care. When appropriate, you should explain to family members how they can support the client's care. If you believe you see any problems with the client's care because of family reasons, you should report them to your supervisor.

It is important to remember that, although you have entered the client's home, you are not a member of the client's family. Do not participate in family disputes. Report problems to your supervisor.

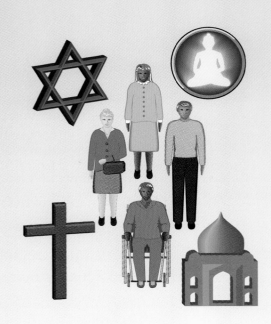

RELIGION & CULTURE

Religion and culture are important issues for almost every client. They provide a sense of security, purpose, and meaning. They also create habits and ways of looking at life that become a basic part of the client's identity. As a result, clients may have strong beliefs about:

- diet;
- clothing;
- personal hygiene;
- sex;
- health care;
- illness;
- death.

Home care aides must accept and respect such beliefs and practices and help clients to find satisfaction in these areas.

Any disrespect of a client's religious and cultural beliefs or practices can be seen as a severe personal insult. If you believe a client's religious or cultural practices are interfering with his or her care, report it to your supervisor.

Aging

Aging is a natural physical process.

After the human body matures, it begins the process of aging. Many physical abilities and functions slowly weaken. If they weaken enough, everyday activities become difficult and severe health problems can occur. Natural wear and tear adds to this process.

Aging has social, psychological, and other elements.

Friends and loved ones die. Social and family roles may change. Retirement from work may be necessary. Health problems increase, become more severe, and can force changes in life style.

The loss of independence can be especially difficult.

As people age, they may need support they didn't need before: to brush their teeth, go to the bathroom, pay their bills, feel appreciated, etc. Depending on others for help can be emotionally difficult. If someone is used to taking care of others, it can be even more difficult.

Each person's experience of aging is different.

For many people, aging is a positive and fulfilling process. For others, it is difficult, frustrating, and painful. Home care aides must act with care, sensitivity, and respect toward each client and treat each one as an individual.

PHYSICAL EFFECTS OF AGING

The most obvious physical changes are to a person's appearance. However, there are many other changes which happen. These often result in loss of ability or function, including*:

- confusion and memory problems;
- poor vision;
- bones that break more easily;
- skin that injures more easily;
- weak muscles;
- less resistance to illness;
- problems with bowel movements and urination;
- heart problems.

see unit 5 for more information on the physical effects of aging.

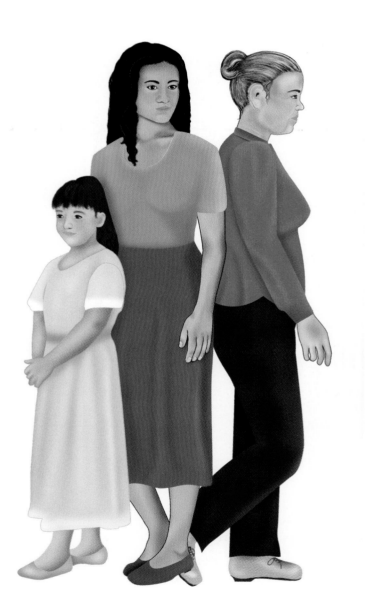

NEED SATISFACTION

The elderly need satisfaction as much as the young. No matter how dependent they may become, the elderly still have a need for esteem and self-actualization.

Home care aides must treat elderly clients in a way that helps them to satisfy their needs and feel good about themselves.

Death and Dying

Most people do not think very often about the fact that they will die. However, it is a very real concern for anyone who is elderly or who has a *terminal illness* (illness that results in death). Since that is true of many clients of home care agencies, coming to terms with death and dying is necessary for home care aides.

STAGES OF DYING

Dr. Elizabeth Kübler-Ross described the emotional process of facing death in five stages:

denial ➤ anger and rage ➤ bargaining ➤ depression ➤ acceptance

No two people face death in the same way, but most will experience some or all of these feelings. Ideally, the dying person will learn to accept death as a natural part of life. However, not everyone does. Some people never get beyond denial or anger. Others believe they can postpone death by bargaining with God. These are normal feelings that must be accepted and respected by home care aides.

HELPING THE DYING PERSON

People who are dying may fear physical pain, worry about family and friends, worry about being a burden, feel sorrow at things they've done, and so on. Some people will not want to discuss these feelings. Others will. If they want to express these feelings, they need to be able to do so openly.

Home care aides must honor and respect those feelings and should be prepared to:

- listen to the person;
- accept his or her feelings about death without judgment;
- make the person as physically comfortable as possible;
- help the person to practice religion or meet with clergy;
- be sensitive to the feelings of the person's family and friends;
- honor as many of the person's wishes as possible.

Some people decide that they do not want to have extraordinary means used to keep them alive or to revive them when they die. They may have a "living will" developed that provides for this. When a dying person should not be revived, *do not resuscitate (DNR)* orders are issued.

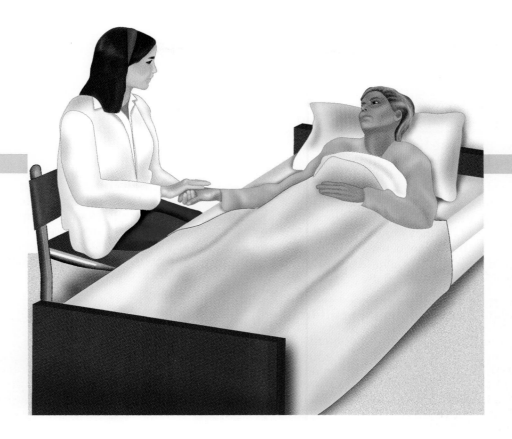

DEATH

Physical signs that death is near include when:

- eyesight dims;
- speech becomes difficult;
- hands and feet become cold;
- skin becomes pale;
- breathing becomes irregular;
- muscles become limp (the jaw may drop).

The dying person can usually hear well. So use a calm and gentle voice. Make the dying person as comfortable as possible.

CARE AFTER DEATH

Postmortem care is care after death. Home care aides may prepare the body of the deceased for viewing by the family or for transfer to a funeral home. This includes placing the deceased on his or her back, removing soiled clothing and dressings, bathing the body, putting on a clean gown, and closing the deceased's eyes. Always use a gentle touch as the body after death is easily bruised. Procedures can differ by agency. You must follow your agency's procedures.

FAMILY

The person's family may have strong feelings about his or her death. It's important you acknowledge these feelings and respect them.

Showing respect for the person and for the family will generally be of more comfort than anything you can say.

Children

Children have the same basic needs as adults but also have special needs.

Children depend either partially or completely upon adults for their health and well-being. Beyond physiological support, they need emotional support, reassurance, and comfort. As they grow older, children (particularly adolescents) become increasingly independent regarding physiological needs but are often significantly dependent emotionally.

Nutrition is especially important in children.

It has a direct effect on growth and development. Infants have special nutritional needs which you should discuss with your supervisor. Children of other ages need a balanced diet (see pages 128-133).

There are special procedures for working with small children.

Many nursing procedures must be adapted to the size and development of the small child. If you will be working with small children, check with your supervisor about special procedures. You must also remember to be simple, direct, and patient in communicating with small children, since their ability to communicate is limited.

As an adult, you will perform an important role in the home.

Children will view you as an adult and may expect you to provide physical and emotional care normally provided by parents or other care-givers. Remember that you are not a family member and must not join in family debates or arguments. You also **cannot punish** children for unacceptable behavior. Discuss with your supervisor any behavior problems that parents or other care-givers cannot handle **and report any signs of abuse or neglect in the home.**

INFANTS

The first year of life is the period of fastest growth and development. It is also a period of **complete dependency** and requires special care and attention. If you are to provide care for an infant, make sure you review all aspects of care with your supervisor.

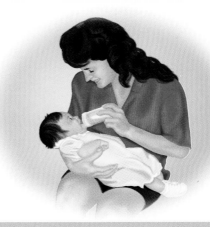

Some guidelines for working with infants:

- ✔ Always support the head and neck of young infants.
- ✔ Burp young infants regularly, either over the shoulder or while sitting on your knee.
- ✔ Change diapers before they are saturated and after bowel movements.
- ✔ Observe stool. It should be a tan color and soft. Report diarrhea immediately—it can cause serious problems.
- ✔ Never leave infants unattended on any surface from which they can fall.
- ✔ Never leave infants unattended in *any* amount of bath water.
- ✔ Keep infants warm (65°-70° room temperature).

mature: fully developed or grown.

TODDLERS

From age 1 to 3, children begin to communicate and develop many physical skills. They are curious and like to explore but they are still largely dependent upon adults. This dependency and curiosity can present safety problems. **If toddlers are present, you will have to take special safety precautions.** Follow your agency's policy for making the home safe *(child-proofing)*.

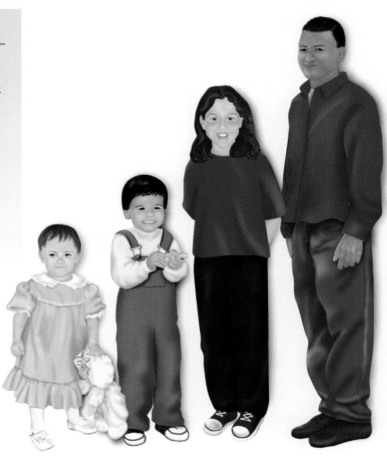

PRE-SCHOOLERS

Pre-schoolers (ages 4 and 5) are active and energetic and can be difficult to watch. However, they can communicate and reason better than toddlers and can begin to assume small amounts of responsibility. Pre-schoolers are prone to getting common colds and the flu. It is important to have good habits of health and hygiene.

SCHOOL-AGE

With the coming of school-age (6-12 years), children are introduced to a powerful environment outside the home. Teachers, friends, and sometimes older children become important influences. Educational difficulties can be a problem. So can sexual development and awareness.

ADOLESCENTS

Adolescence (13-19 years) is a period of rapid sexual development and increasing physical maturity. It is also a period of great emotional stress and conflict as children try to deal with the coming of adulthood. Adolescents generally seek the approval of their peers—friends and other adolescents—over adults.

Behavior

A person's needs are shown in his or her behavior.

When their needs are satisfied, people will generally show positive behavior. When not satisfied, they may show negative behavior as a result of their drive to become satisfied.

"Difficult" clients are usually showing the difficulty they feel over their condition.

The ill, disabled, and elderly often display negative behavior such as argumentativeness, aggression, depression, fear, and lack of cooperation. It may be the only way they feel they can respond to their inability to satisfy their needs.

The health care process is psychological as well as physiological for clients.

Clients must learn to accept their condition and believe in their care. They have to become involved in their care and willing to work toward its success. Depending on the client and the situation, these can be *very* difficult psychological steps to take.

However a client behaves, the home care aide must respond appropriately.

You will have to find ways to control any urges to respond negatively to clients that anger you. A calm and caring response to negative client behavior should have a positive effect on the situation and may help you to improve the client's behavior. Report negative behavior to your supervisor. Your supervisor may be able to both help you deal with the client *and* find ways to improve the client's behavior.

APPROPRIATE

- ✔ Cooperation
- ✔ Courtesy
- ✔ Responsibility

CLIENT BEHAVIOR

NOT APPROPRIATE

- ✘ Argumentativeness
- ✘ Rudeness
- ✘ Aggression
- ✘ Lack of cooperation

The home care aide needs to identify and understand client behavior and respond appropriately.

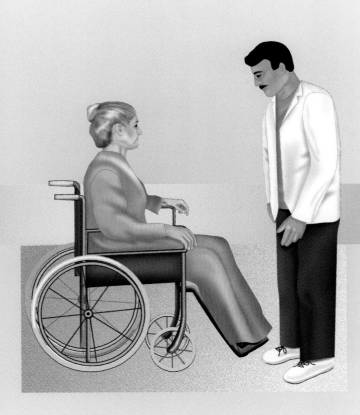

APPROPRIATE

✔ **Acceptance**

✔ **Courtesy**

✔ **Empathy**

✔ **Patience**

✔ **Support**

AIDE RESPONSE

NOT APPROPRIATE

✘ **Rudeness**

✘ **Criticism**

✘ **Neglect**

✘ **Abuse**

✘ **Sarcasm**

☞ *It's natural to get angry at clients sometimes. It's just not acceptable to take it out on them. Talk with your supervisor about how you can respond correctly to the situation.*

Client Needs & Behavior

1.
Imagine a friend or family member becomes a client of a home care agency . How would you like him or her to be treated by the agency's home care aides?

2.
Consider all the aspects of becoming elderly (the loss of friends, illness, etc.) that you would find difficult. List what you believe would be the five most difficult for you to accept.

3.
If you knew you were dying, what would you want to do or have?

4.
There are many ways to control anger (taking a time-out, exercise, etc.). Think of examples where people have made you angry and you have let them know it. How would you have been able to let out your anger in other ways?

REVIEW

**Key Terms – Test your understanding of each of these first.
Then use each one once to fill in the incomplete statements below.**

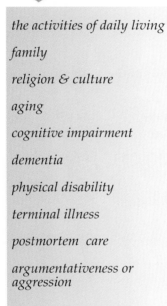

the activities of daily living

family

religion & culture

aging

cognitive impairment

dementia

physical disability

terminal illness

postmortem care

argumentativeness or aggression

1. Physiologically caused cognitive impairment which gets progressively worse until all cognitive ability is lost is called _____ .

2. You must not respond to negative client behavior such as _____ by showing anger at the client.

3. Denial, anger, and depression are common responses to _____.

4. _____ causes many physical abilities and functions to slowly weaken, making everyday activities difficult to perform.

5. _____ relationships are often the most meaningful parts of a person's life.

6. Assistive devices can help clients with a _____ perform self-care that would otherwise be impossible.

7. _____ is care after death.

8. _____ create habits and ways of looking at life that must be accepted and respected by home care aides.

9. _____ is the inability to understand, remember, or think in normal ways.

10. Providing as much self-care as possible for _____ _____ helps clients' feelings of independence and self-esteem.

The Body's System

A system is a set of things which work together as one.

The human body is a system of systems. Organs are made up of tissues. Tissues are made up of cells. Cells are made up of molecules (like water or proteins). They work together to form the body's system.

The body's major systems are its organ systems.

These systems perform functions like protection, motion, and control. They are grouped at right by their main function. In addition to these functions, the systems often perform other important functions and overlap.

Any system has a condition at which it functions best.

The physical and chemical processes by which the body's system functions are called its *metabolism.* *Homeostasis* is the condition in which the metabolism stays at a level that allows the body to function best. Disease weakens the body's ability to maintain homeostasis. This causes changes in temperature, pulse, etc., which are called *symptoms*.

The body's systems depend on each other.

Like the systems of an automobile (engine, transmission, etc.), the systems of the body work together to keep the body functioning normally. When one system doesn't work correctly, it affects other systems and may cause them to not work correctly either. If the problem of one system is serious enough, it can lead to death.

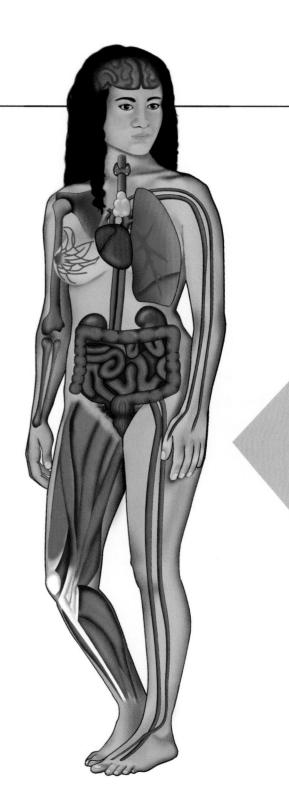

Anatomy: The structure of a body or organism.

Physiology: The way a body works. Its functions and processes.

STRUCTURE, MOTION, PROTECTION

- **Integumentary System (Skin):** Shields the body's systems from disease or injury, and helps to control temperature.

- **Skeletal System:** Provides structure, protects key organs, and stores minerals.

- **Muscular System:** Protects soft tissue, produces heat, and enables motion.

INTAKE AND OUTPUT

- **Respiratory System:** Takes in oxygen, releases carbon dioxide gas (waste).

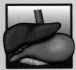
- **Digestive System:** Takes in nutrients, absorbs them for the body's use, and eliminates solid waste.

- **Urinary System:** Eliminates waste fluids.

CONTROL

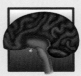
- **Nervous System:** Receives and processes information and regulates the body's response.

- **Endocrine System:** Releases hormones which regulate many system functions.

CIRCULATION

- **Cardiovascular System:** Carries nutrients and oxygen in the blood to cells, and carries waste away.

- **Lymphatic System:** Attacks pathogens and toxins and circulates lymph fluid.

REPRODUCTION

- **Reproductive:** Keeps the species alive by producing children.

The Integumentary System

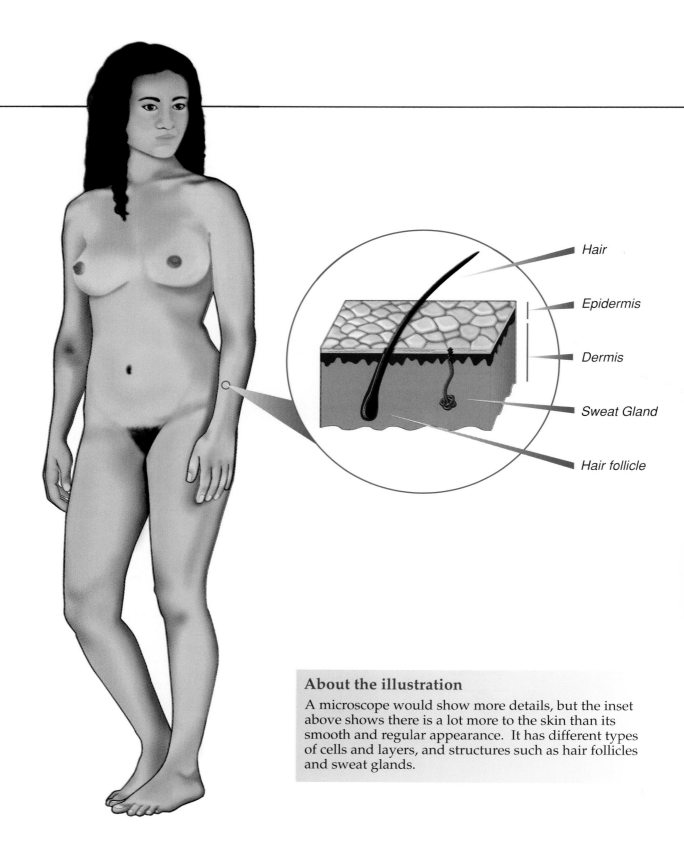

Hair

Epidermis

Dermis

Sweat Gland

Hair follicle

About the illustration

A microscope would show more details, but the inset above shows there is a lot more to the skin than its smooth and regular appearance. It has different types of cells and layers, and structures such as hair follicles and sweat glands.

Overview

- The *integumentary* system (the skin) is made up of two primary layers, the *epidermis* (the surface) and the *dermis* (underneath), with additional structures such as hair, nails, and glands.

- It is the body's first line of defense, acting as a barrier against disease and other hazards.

- It helps control temperature by releasing heat through sweat or by restricting blood vessels to act as insulation.

- It is a primary source of *sensory information,* having nerve endings that are sensitive to pressure, temperature, pleasure and pain.

Disorders

- The skin is a disease warning system. Changes in its color, surface, temperature, and moistness are each possible signs of a problem and require attention.

- *Decubitus ulcers (bedsores* or *pressure sores)* are areas where skin and sometimes the tissue underneath it have died as a result of poor circulation and pressure. This is a common and serious problem for clients confined to bed or who have difficulty moving.

- Burns kill the skin by layer. *First degree* kills the outer layer of the epidermis. *Second degree* kills all layers of the epidermis. *Third degree* kills the epidermis and dermis.

- *Skin cancers* as a result of sun exposure appear as open sores *(lesions)* or discolored areas.

Aging

- The skin thins and loses its ability to stretch *(elasticity),* making it easier to injure.

- Its ability to protect the body against infection and to repair itself weakens.

- It becomes less effective at temperature control.

The Skeletal System

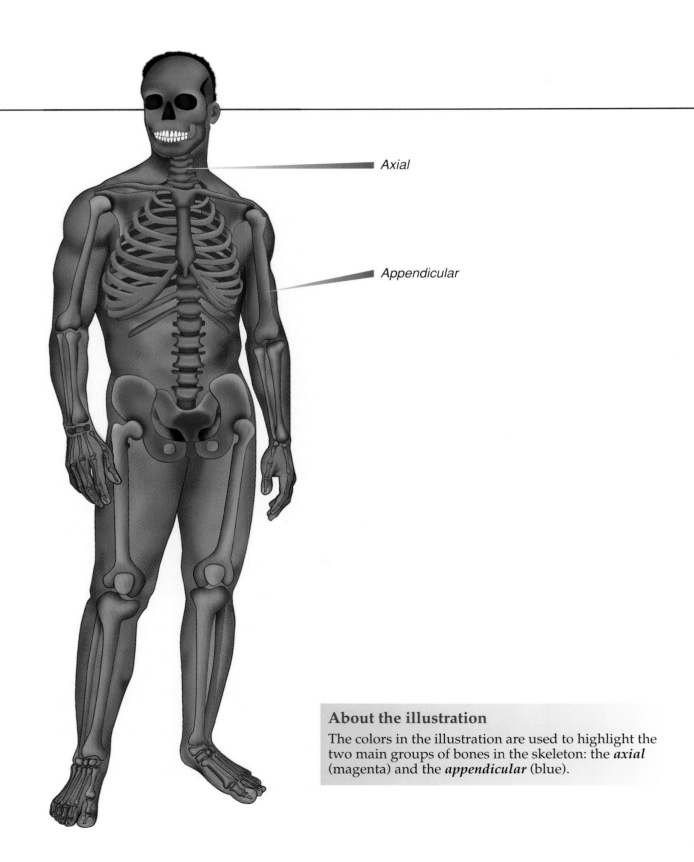

Axial

Appendicular

About the illustration

The colors in the illustration are used to highlight the two main groups of bones in the skeleton: the *axial* (magenta) and the *appendicular* (blue).

Overview

- The *skeletal* system protects soft organs and provides structure and support for the rest of the body's systems. It works together with the muscle system to provide precise and powerful movement.

- Made up largely of hard *osseous* (bone) tissue, it is a living system which undergoes dynamic changes throughout life. It is the body's warehouse for calcium and its factory for red blood cells (produced by *bone marrow*, found inside hollow bones).

- The system's 206 bones are called *axial* (brain & spinal cord) or *appendicular* (arms, legs, and connecting bones). They are held together at joints by connective tissue such as *ligaments* (dense fibers) and *cartilage* (a tough and flexible tissue). Joints range from rigid to those allowing full motion (the ball-in-socket joints of the hip and shoulders).

Disorders

- *Fractures* are breaks in bones. Complete breaks are usually obvious. Incomplete breaks may only be noticeable by a bruise, swelling, or pain when pressure is directly applied.

- *Arthritis* is a disorder of the movable joints that has different forms. It can be very painful and can cause severe joint damage that will limit movement.

- *Bursitis* is a joint disorder caused by repetitive motion. It can be very painful but generally will heal if the cause is discontinued.

Aging

- Beginning in the thirties, bones gradually weaken and shrink (in women faster than men), allowing them to break more easily. *Osteoporosis* is a severe condition of this. It strikes women much more than men.

- Joint cartilage wears out from use. This causes *osteoarthritis* and weakening of the joints.

- The skeletal system becomes more vulnerable to diseases such as *osteomyelitis*.

The Muscular System

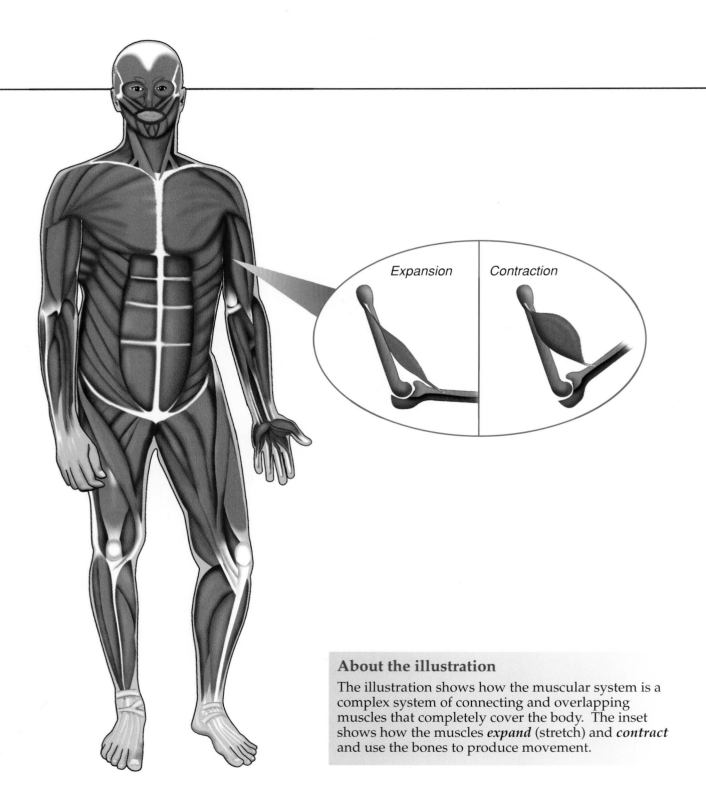

Expansion

Contraction

About the illustration

The illustration shows how the muscular system is a complex system of connecting and overlapping muscles that completely cover the body. The inset shows how the muscles *expand* (stretch) and *contract* and use the bones to produce movement.

Overview

- The muscular system is primarily made up of *skeletal muscles* which attach to the skeleton. These muscles pull and push the bones to cause body movement. This in turn produces heat to keep the body warm.

- The action of most skeletal muscles is called *voluntary* because it is controlled consciously. *Involuntary* muscles operate automatically and are found in the heart, the stomach, or in walls of blood vessels.

- Skeletal muscles protect soft tissues, control the motions of the mouth for eating, cause the breathing action of the lungs, and perform many other important functions.

Disorders

- Minor muscle disorders such as *cramps* or *strains* are common and often the result of a simple cause like too little water *(dehydration)* or too much exercise. Muscles gradually return to normal when the cause is removed.

- Muscles that are not used become smaller and lose strength *(atrophy)*. They can deform into *contractures* (knot-like deformities), causing permanent loss of function. Contractures are a common and serious problem among clients who have difficulty moving. Exercising muscles regularly prevents atrophy and contractures.

- *Muscular dystrophy* is a non-contagious disease which progressively weakens and cripples the muscles and results in death.

Aging

- Muscles gradually lose strength and endurance, beginning in middle age.

- They can develop *fibrosis*, a condition of the muscle fibers which makes them stiffer and less useful.

- Their ability to repair injury weakens.

The Nervous System

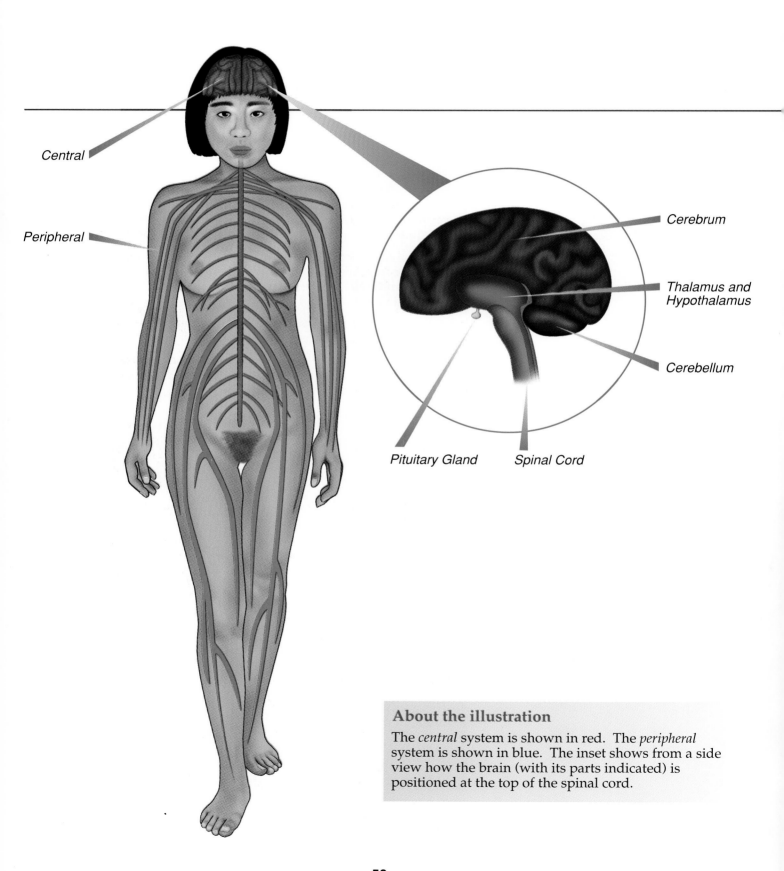

Central

Peripheral

Cerebrum

Thalamus and
Hypothalamus

Cerebellum

Pituitary Gland   Spinal Cord

About the illustration

The *central* system is shown in red. The *peripheral*
system is shown in blue. The inset shows from a side
view how the brain (with its parts indicated) is
positioned at the top of the spinal cord.

Overview

- The *Nervous System* is a communication system. It uses highly specialized *neural tissue* to send and receive information in the form of chemical and electrical signals. When injured, neural tissue generally cannot recover and loses its ability to function.

- The *central nervous system* (made up of the brain and spinal cord) processes *sensory* (sight, taste, etc.) and *motor* (movement) information and regulates the systems of the body.

- The *peripheral nervous* system (consisting of the *cranial* and *spinal nerves)* carries information throughout the body and links the body's systems together.

- Automatic functions of the body (breathing, digestion, etc.) are regulated by the *autonomic nervous system* It includes elements of both the central and peripheral systems.

Disorders

- *Spinal cord injuries* cause temporary or permanent *paralysis* (loss of sensation, motion, and function). A severed or cut spinal cord results in *paraplegia* (paralysis of the legs) or *quadriplegia* (paralysis of the arms *and* legs).

- A *stroke* (cerebrovascular accident) cuts off blood circulation to the brain resulting in loss of sensory and motor skills that can be minor or major.

- *Epilepsy* is a condition of abnormal electrical activity in the brain resulting in convulsions (seizures).

- *Multiple sclerosis* is a crippling disease which gradually destroys the central nervous system, usually over many years.

Aging

- Memory weakens, especially recent *(secondary)* memory. Sensory ability (sight, taste, hearing, etc.) and motor control weaken. Reflexes slow.

- *Alzheimer's disease* primarily affects the elderly. The initial symptom is forgetfulness which progresses to total loss of emotional and intellectual control.

- *Parkinson's disease* affects the elderly more than other age groups. It causes muscle tremors and spastic movement. It can be treated with drugs.

The Endocrine System

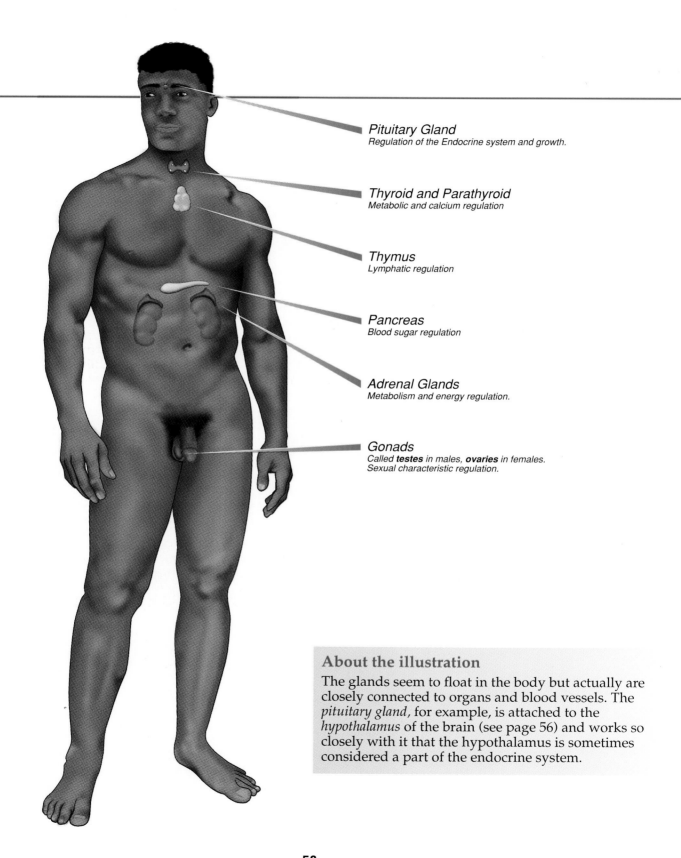

Pituitary Gland
Regulation of the Endocrine system and growth.

Thyroid and Parathyroid
Metabolic and calcium regulation

Thymus
Lymphatic regulation

Pancreas
Blood sugar regulation

Adrenal Glands
Metabolism and energy regulation.

Gonads
Called **testes** in males, **ovaries** in females.
Sexual characteristic regulation.

About the illustration

The glands seem to float in the body but actually are closely connected to organs and blood vessels. The *pituitary gland*, for example, is attached to the *hypothalamus* of the brain (see page 56) and works so closely with it that the hypothalamus is sometimes considered a part of the endocrine system.

Overview

- The endocrine system is the body's chemical system of control. It works closely with the nervous system to control homeostasis and body functions. Its specialized organs (called *glands)* produce chemicals (called *hormones)* which regulate growth, blood sugar, metabolism, reproduction, and other processes.

- The *pituitary gland* controls the body's growth and releases hormones into the bloodstream which control much of the activity of the other glands. It is controlled by hormones released by the *hypothalamus* of the brain (see page 56).

- Abnormal hormone amounts in the body or abnormal tissue sensitivity to hormones hurts the body's ability to function and can have serious results.

Disorders

- *Diabetes mellitus* is a disorder in which the *pancreas* does not produce enough *insulin* hormone to allow the body to use blood sugar. It can damage the cardiovascular and nervous systems and lead to strokes, *gangrene* (death of tissue due to lack of circulation), and death. Early symptoms are increased thirst and urination. Severe cases are called *insulin dependent* and require insulin injections.

- *Hyperthyroidism* from an overactive thyroid causes a very high metabolic rate and such symptoms as nervousness and weight loss. *Hypothyroidism* from an underactive thyroid causes poor physical and mental development.

Aging

- The body's tissues become less sensitive to hormones, which weakens their effectiveness.

- Levels of the reproductive hormones (*androgens* for males and estrogens for females) lower. A lowering in estrogen levels in women is associated with *menopause* (page 71) and with osteoporosis (page 53). Elderly men have lower levels of *testosterone*, an androgen, which may result in less sexual activity.

The Cardiovascular System

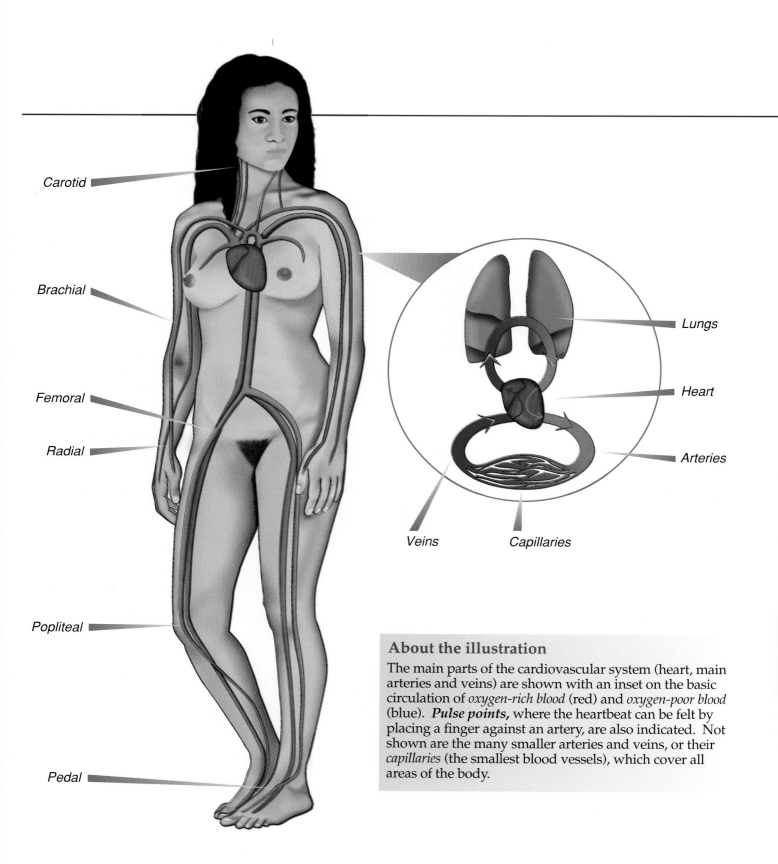

Carotid

Brachial

Femoral

Radial

Popliteal

Pedal

Lungs

Heart

Arteries

Veins

Capillaries

About the illustration

The main parts of the cardiovascular system (heart, main arteries and veins) are shown with an inset on the basic circulation of *oxygen-rich blood* (red) and *oxygen-poor blood* (blue). ***Pulse points,*** where the heartbeat can be felt by placing a finger against an artery, are also indicated. Not shown are the many smaller arteries and veins, or their *capillaries* (the smallest blood vessels), which cover all areas of the body.

Overview

- The *cardiovascular* or *circulatory system* distributes blood and all it carries throughout the body: nutrients and oxygen to cells for energy; waste and toxins away for elimination; heat to maintain temperature; hormones for regulation; antibodies that fight disease; etc.

- The heart pumps oxygen-rich blood from the lungs (see inset at left) into *arteries* for distribution to the body. After it is used, oxygen-poor blood returns through capillaries into veins and back to the heart and lungs.

- Blood is made up of a liquid *(plasma)* that has cellular material *(blood cells and platelets)* suspended in it. *Red blood cells* carry oxygen and carbon dioxide. *White blood cells* fight infection. *Platelets* close wounds by thickening *(clotting)* the blood.

Disorders

- *Anemia* is a disorder that results in a low level of oxygen in the blood and loss of energy or strength. It can have many causes and treatments.

- *Hypertension* is abnormally high blood pressure caused by blocked arteries that force the heart to work harder to pump blood through the body. Over time, this can cause serious damage to the heart and blood vessels.

- Blocked coronary arteries in the heart supply less blood to heart muscle. If the blockages are severe enough, muscle tissue dies and a *heart attack (myocardial infarction)* occurs, which can cause death.

Aging

- The heart weakens and becomes easier to damage.

- *Ateriosclerosis* thickens and stiffens artery walls. This affects blood supply and can cause serious damage or death.

- Circulation weakens, allowing water to be retained, dangerous blood clots to form more easily, and the weakening of many of the body's functions.

The Lymphatic System

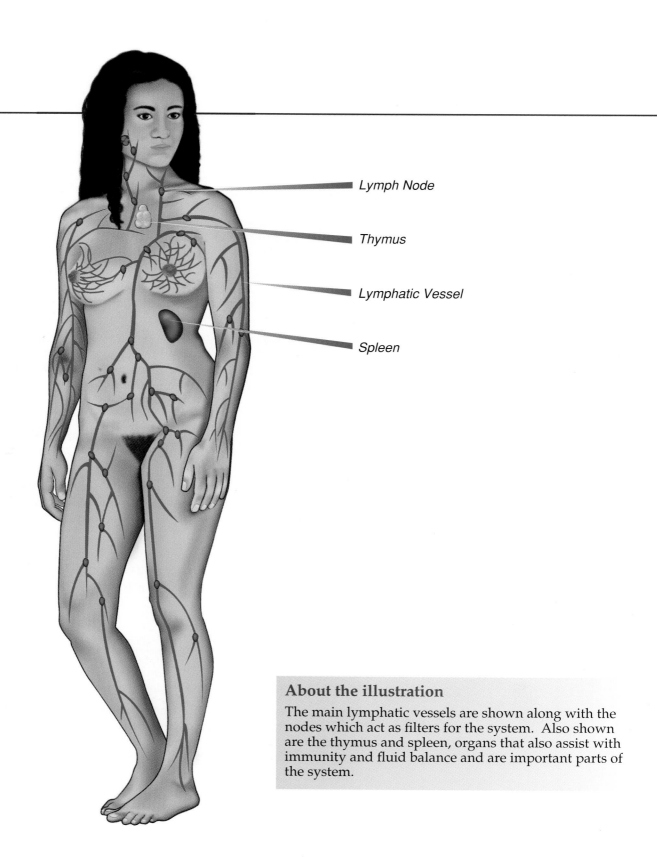

Lymph Node

Thymus

Lymphatic Vessel

Spleen

About the illustration

The main lymphatic vessels are shown along with the nodes which act as filters for the system. Also shown are the thymus and spleen, organs that also assist with immunity and fluid balance and are important parts of the system.

Overview

- The lymphatic system (like the cardiovascular system with which it works closely) circulates fluid to help control homeostasis throughout the body. Fluid from body tissues *(lymph)* flows into a network of *lymphatic vessels* where it is filtered for impurities by *lymph nodes* (small round organs).

- The lymphatic system is the center of the body's *immune system*. It contains large amounts of *lymphocytes* (a type of white blood cell) that attack disease. Lymphocytes release *antibodies* that destroy disease cells, providing *immunity* (a barrier to disease).

- The *tonsils, spleen*, and *thymus* are lymphatic organs that help fluid balance and immunity outside the network of lymphatic vessels. The spleen, for example, filters the blood much the way the nodes filter lymph.

Disorders

- *Allergies* are an immune response to foreign substances like pollen or chemicals. Most are not severe. However, some allergies (to a drug or bee sting, for example) can cause serious reactions.

- When lymphocytes collect in a node to fight infection, the node often swells as a noticeable symptom. This is true for many common infections but also applies to possibly fatal ones such as *lymphoma*, cancer of the lymph nodes.

- The *HIV* virus causes *Acquired Immune Deficiency Syndrome (AIDS)*. AIDS destroys the immune system's ability to defend the body against infection and results in death.

Aging

- The body's immunity to pathogens gradually weakens, making it easier to become infected. As a result, *vaccines* (substances that increase immunity) are often ordered for the elderly, especially as protection against common infections like the flu.

- It is generally believed that the immune system successfully attacks cancer cells throughout most of life but that the ability to fight cancer cells weakens in the elderly. They have a higher rate of cancer than people of other ages.

The Respiratory System

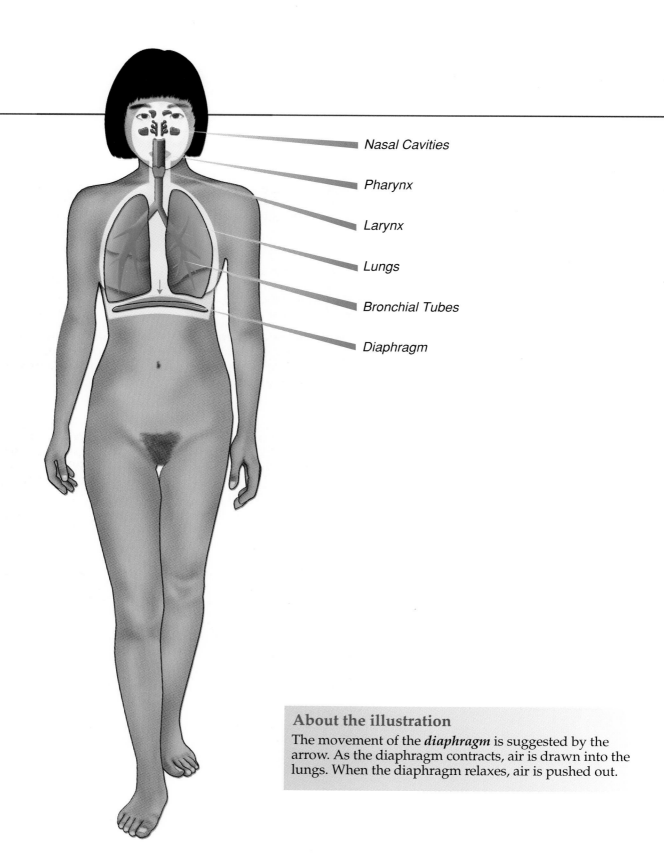

Nasal Cavities

Pharynx

Larynx

Lungs

Bronchial Tubes

Diaphragm

About the illustration

The movement of the *diaphragm* is suggested by the arrow. As the diaphragm contracts, air is drawn into the lungs. When the diaphragm relaxes, air is pushed out.

Overview

- *The cells of the body need oxygen to live.* It is their source of energy. The use of oxygen produces *carbon dioxide* waste. The respiratory system allows the body to take in oxygen from the air and to send out carbon dioxide. It produces sound for speaking and also helps to cool the body.

- The *respiratory muscles* (especially the *diaphragm*) expand the lungs automatically, causing air to be inhaled through the *upper respiratory tract (nasal cavities, pharynx, larynx* and *trachea)*. These passageways partially filter and warm the air for the *lungs*.

- The lungs use special tissue called *alveoli* to transfer oxygen into the blood and carbon dioxide out of the lungs. The respiratory muscles squeeze the lungs, forcing out the air with the carbon dioxide in it.

Disorders

- The respiratory system can be infected by many contagious diseases. *Common colds, flu, pneumonia,* and *tuberculosis* can be caused by inhaling pathogens sneezed or coughed into the air by an infected person. Pneumonia and tuberculosis are severe infections of the lungs that can cause death if not treated.

- A *pulmonary embolism* is a blockage of a lung artery by a blood clot. It can collapse a lung and cause the heart to fail from the extra strain.

- *Lung cancer* is a highly fatal cancer related to cigarette smoking. However, if smoking is stopped soon enough, lung damage can be reversed and the risk of cancer reduced.

Aging

- The ability of the lungs to take in air and then absorb oxygen weakens. This weakens the body's ability to produce energy.

- Circulatory problems from aging increase the possibility of blood clotting and a pulmonary embolism forming.

The Digestive System

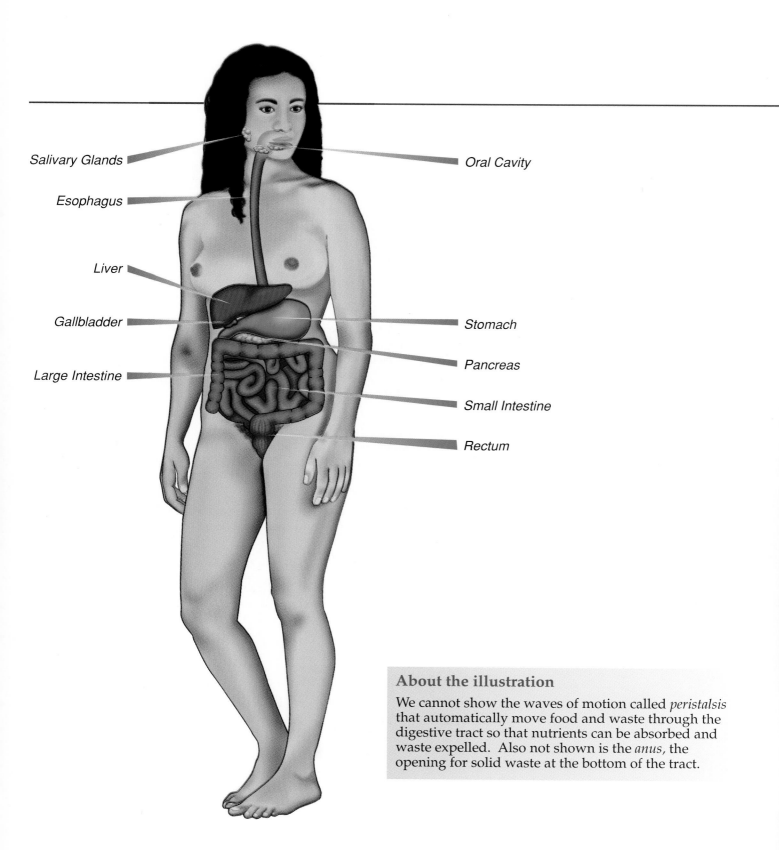

Salivary Glands

Esophagus

Liver

Gallbladder

Large Intestine

Oral Cavity

Stomach

Pancreas

Small Intestine

Rectum

About the illustration

We cannot show the waves of motion called *peristalsis* that automatically move food and waste through the digestive tract so that nutrients can be absorbed and waste expelled. Also not shown is the *anus*, the opening for solid waste at the bottom of the tract.

Overview

- The digestive system: 1.) takes in food *(ingestion)*; 2.) takes out nutrients and water from it *(digestion)*; 3.) transfers them to the body's systems *(absorption)*; and 4.) disposes of what it doesn't need as waste *(excretion)*.

- It is made up of the *digestive tract* (oral cavity, esophagus, stomach, small intestine, and large intestine) and *accessory organs* (salivary glands, liver, pancreas, and gallbladder). The accessory organs produce chemicals called *enzymes* that break down food into nutrients and waste.

- The stomach breaks food down for digestion using powerful acids and enzymes. The small intestine absorbs nutrients and water into the body. The large intestine absorbs excess water into the body and eliminates *feces* (solid waste) and *flatus* (gaseous waste) out the *rectum* and *anus*.

Disorders

- *Diarrhea* causes normally solid feces to become more liquid. Generally caused by viruses or bacteria, it can cause serious problems if not treated.

- *Peritonitis* is an infection of intestinal lining from appendicitis, ruptured ulcers, or wounds that can lead to death.

- *Ulcers* are areas where intestinal lining has been damaged, exposing tissue to intestinal acids. Burning pain is a common symptom, blood in the feces a more dangerous symptom.

- *Hepatitis* is a disease that attacks the liver. Depending on the type (A, B, C, D, or E), infection can come from ingestion of fecally (feces) contaminated material or be blood-borne.

Aging

- Irregular bowel movement *(constipation)* increases as intestinal muscles weaken from aging. Generally, diet and exercise are the best response. Enemas and laxatives should be used only as prescribed by a physician.

- Ulcers form more easily as the stomach lining weakens.

- Cancers increase, especially colon and stomach cancer.

The Urinary System

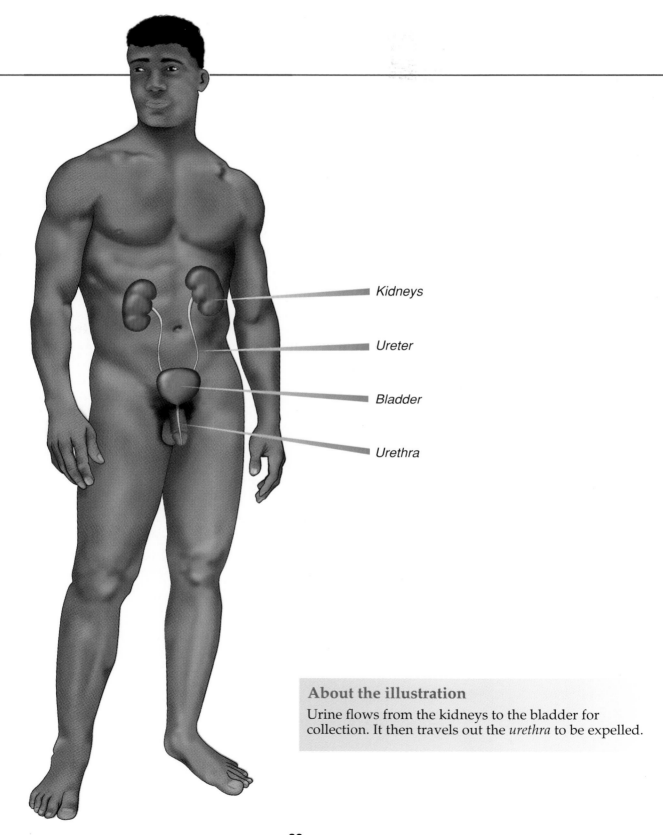

Kidneys

Ureter

Bladder

Urethra

About the illustration

Urine flows from the kidneys to the bladder for collection. It then travels out the *urethra* to be expelled.

Overview

- The average person takes in and puts out the same amount of water daily—about 2.5 liters. Of this, about one liter is put out as *urine,* the waste-carrying water produced by the urinary system.

- *Kidneys* filter the blood for unwanted material and make urine. This liquid waste then flows down the *ureters* to the *bladder* for collection. Once enough urine is collected, the body automatically urges itself to eliminate it.

- In eliminating waste, the urinary system helps control the body's fluid balance and *acid-base balance (pH).* (Too much fluid or too much change in pH can cause death.) It also helps control blood pressure.

Disorders

- *Cystitis* and *urethritis* are infections of the urinary system with symptoms of frequent and painful (often burning) urination. Women are more likely than men to develop cystitis.

- *Kidney disease* is any of a number of conditions (often resulting from an infection) which damage the kidney. If severe, it can cause the kidney to stop working *(renal failure).* Common symptoms are *edema* (too much retention of water) or *dehydration* (too much output of water in the urine).

Aging

- The kidneys become less efficient at producing urine, requiring a greater daily intake of water.

- Automatic bladder control often weakens, causing involuntary leaking of urine *(incontinence).*

- The body's defense against kidney disease weakens.

The Reproductive System

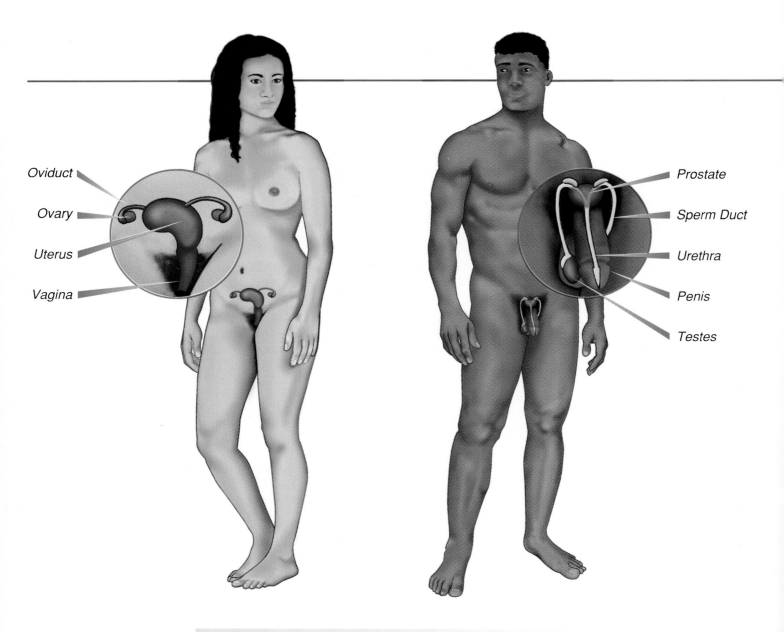

Oviduct

Ovary

Uterus

Vagina

Prostate

Sperm Duct

Urethra

Penis

Testes

About the illustration

Compared to the other systems or to how important it is, the area devoted to reproduction is relatively small. Not shown are the even smaller sperm and eggs which cause reproduction. Each egg travels down tubes from the ovaries to the uterus. Once sperm from the male is placed in the female vagina, it will also travel to the uterus to fertilize the egg.

Overview

- The *reproductive system* keeps the species alive. Male and female systems differ but work together *sexually* to produce children. The male's *penis* and the female's *vagina* are called *genitals*. The penis fits into the vagina to allow reproduction to happen.

- The female's ovaries produce an *ova* (egg). The male's *testes* produce *spermatozoa* (sperm). Each contains half the reproductive material *(chromosomes)* necessary for life. The sperm and ova join (the act of *fertilization*) in the female's uterus to form an *embryo*. It will develop into an infant over approximately 280 days.

- The female's uterus is prepared for this on a monthly basis by the collection of nutrient-rich blood in its lining *(endometrium)*. If there is no fertilization, the uterus sheds the blood, lining, and unfertilized egg in the process of *menstruation.*

Disorders

- *Infertility* or *sterility* is the inability to reproduce. It affects both sexes and can be complete or partial.

- *Venereal diseases* are diseases spread by sexual contact. Gonorrhea, syphilis, herpes, and genital warts are among the most common types. They affect both sexes.

- Infections and tumors of the uterus are common problems for women. When severe, they can cause sterility. A *hysterectomy* is the surgical removal of the uterus.

Aging

- Production of sperm in males steadily becomes less in the adult years until it ends. The ovaries of women stop functioning after mid-life and the menstrual cycle stops completely *(menopause)*.

- Less hormones are produced, affecting sexual characteristics and activity.

- Rate of *breast cancer* in women increases. *Prostate* infections and cancers in men increase.

Anatomy and Physiology

1.

Think of a system with which you are familiar (transit, political, legal, etc.). What makes that system work poorly or well? Can you make any comparisons to the body's system?

2.

Which of your body's systems are you most aware of? Why? Do you think this is true of most people? Why?

3.

Make a list of ten observable signs that a body is not functioning as it should.

4.

List the physical results of aging that you feel will be most difficult for you to accept.

REVIEW

**Key Terms – Test your understanding of each of these first.
Then use each one once to fill in the incomplete statements below.**

homeostasis

epidermis

dermis

osseous tissue

atrophy

neural tissue

hormones

red blood cells

immunity

oxygen

absorption

feces

urine

chromosomes

fertilization

1. _____ (bone) is the body's warehouse for calcium.

2. Chemicals called _____ perform much of the body's regulation.

3. _____ are solid wastes produced in the large intestine. _____ is liquid waste produced in the kidneys.

4. _____ is the condition in which the metabolism stays at a level that allows the body to function best.

5. Muscles that are not used will shrink in size and strength (_____).

6. _____ carry oxygen and carbon dioxide.

7. _____ can send and receive information in the form of chemical and electrical signals.

8. The _____ of males and females contain half the genetic information necessary for life. _____ is when sperm and egg join in the female's uterus.

9. _____ is required by the body's cells to produce the energy they need to function.

10. Lymphocytes produce antibodies that provide _____ to disease.

11. The _____ is the surface layer of skin and the _____ lies underneath.

12. After food is broken down in digestion, nutrients are transferred to the body's systems through the process of _____ .

Care of the Home

You will be trusted to be alone with clients in their homes.

You must respect and safeguard your clients' personal property. This includes everything in the home *and* money. It's against the law to damage or steal a client's personal property.

You will perform housekeeping, laundry, and shopping services for clients.

Many clients need help to maintain their home. You may be expected to perform light cleaning, wash linens and other laundry, buy groceries, etc. Your agency will indicate the activities you are to perform on the client's care plan, activity sheet, or other written form. **Only perform the activities your agency indicates to you in writing.**

Your goal is to provide the client with a safe, clean, and pleasant environment.

This is necessary for good health care and will help clients feel better about themselves *and* you. If clients see that you respect and care for their home, they will be more cooperative. You will also feel more comfortable working in such an environment. To maintain this environment, you will need to perform many activities routinely.

You must respect the client's home just as you respect the client.

The client's home is a reflection of the client. Disrespect of the home may be seen as a severe personal insult. You must also honor any habits, preferences, or rules for activities in the home (including housekeeping) that clients may have.

Your agency will indicate in writing the activities you are to perform in each client's home. Accommodate each client's preferences as much as possible while following agency guidelines. Report any unusual requests or conditions to your supervisor.

An environment that meets clients' basic needs is necessary for good health care. See pages 32-33.

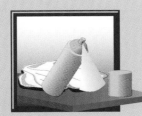

HOUSEKEEPING

You may perform light housekeeping for some clients. This means keeping the home neat and clean. It does not mean any activities requiring heavy lifting, climbing, using unusually harsh chemicals, etc. When in doubt, check with your supervisor.

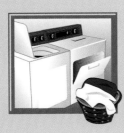

LAUNDRY

It is important to keep linens and clothing fresh, both for health and personal reasons. You will need to know how to handle different types of laundry since some need special handling. You may also be given special instructions regarding handling laundry of clients with infectious disorders.

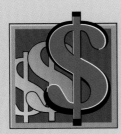

SHOPPING & MONEY MANAGEMENT

Some clients will need you to perform shopping, banking, or other activities involving money. This is a great responsibility and an area for potential conflict. You will be required to carefully account for all money handled and to make sure that clients get what they need at prices they should pay.

Housekeeping

Maintaining a clean and neat home takes planning and regular upkeep. Because there are many different tasks in housekeeping, it is important to have a *housekeeping plan* to keep track of everything. Some tasks need to be performed daily; some weekly; some several times a week; and so on. You will use different types of equipment and cleaning products and must make sure you have them when you need them.

A housekeeping plan will help you keep track of housekeeping tasks and the equipment and supplies needed to perform them. Remember that you are only to perform the activities that are indicated to you in writing by your supervisor. Clients and family members will be expected to perform the other tasks.

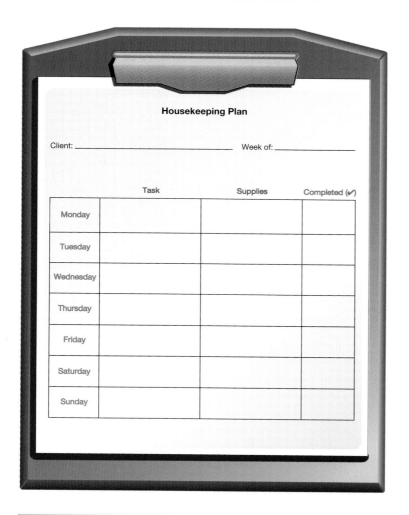

Housekeeping Plan

Client: _____   Week of: _____

	Task	Supplies	Completed (✔)
Monday			
Tuesday			
Wednesday			
Thursday			
Friday			
Saturday			
Sunday			

✔ Use your plan to **check** that you have all the supplies and equipment you need **before you start.**

A clean and neat home creates a safe environment for health care. Cleaning prevents the spread of germs, protects food from spoiling, etc. Keeping a neat or orderly home also contributes to safety: floors are not cluttered; medications are where they need to be; dangerous chemicals are stored; etc.

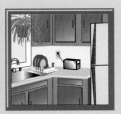

KITCHEN

It is essential that the kitchen be a safe and pleasant room since it is where food is prepared, stored, and (depending upon the home) eaten—among the most basic of human needs. Note that there are important safety issues in every kitchen regarding food spoilage and fire.

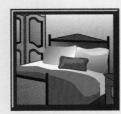

BEDROOM

All clients spend a great deal of time in their bedrooms, even if only to sleep. For clients undergoing bedrest, the bedroom becomes the central room of their home. It is important to make beds regularly, keep linens clean, and to maintain a clean and neat room.

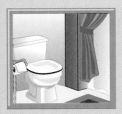

BATHROOM

Many accidents occur in the bathroom and many germs are spread there as well. Maintaining a clean and neat bathroom is necessary to personal hygiene, safety, and infection control.

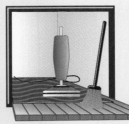

FLOORS & CARPETS

Floors need to be free for walking. They should be regularly swept and mopped if bare, or vacuumed if carpeted or covered with rugs.

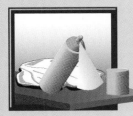

DUSTING

Dusty surfaces are unattractive and can aggravate allergies. Dusting is light work best performed with a soft cloth and a dust spray.

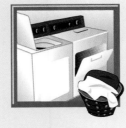

LAUNDRY

Clean clothes and linens are necessary for a clean home and for personal hygiene and grooming. You may receive special laundry instructions for clients with infectious disorders.

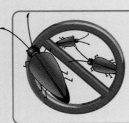

PESTS

Pests (roaches, mice, etc.) can carry infection, damage property, and cause other problems. Keeping surfaces clean, disposing of garbage regularly, and maintaining a neat and clean home will help prevent this. You may also need to use pest control chemicals or devices.

Kitchen

Kitchens must be kept clean and neat for safe meal preparation (see page 137 on **Food Safety**) and they should be a pleasant room in which to eat. Because kitchens are so important and are used so much, they require constant attention. Each meal requires clean-up, and many activities must be performed daily.

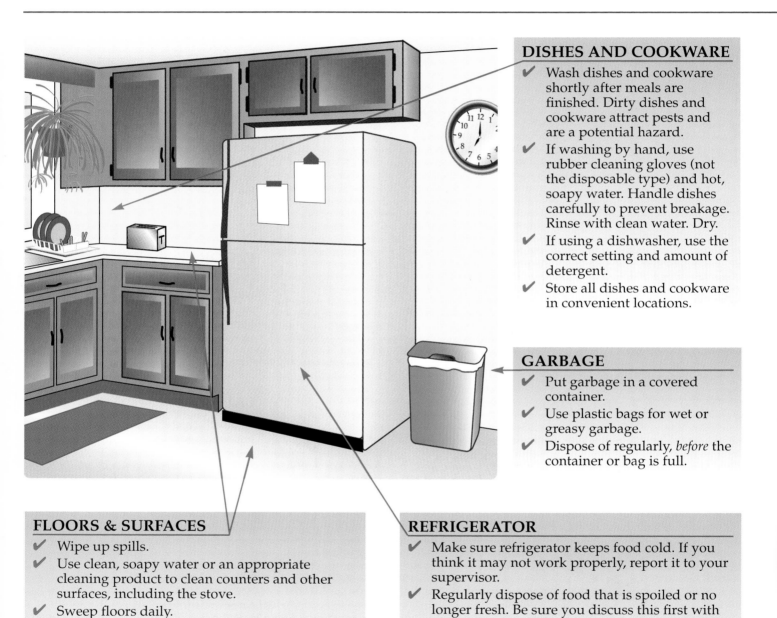

DISHES AND COOKWARE

✔ Wash dishes and cookware shortly after meals are finished. Dirty dishes and cookware attract pests and are a potential hazard.

✔ If washing by hand, use rubber cleaning gloves (not the disposable type) and hot, soapy water. Handle dishes carefully to prevent breakage. Rinse with clean water. Dry.

✔ If using a dishwasher, use the correct setting and amount of detergent.

✔ Store all dishes and cookware in convenient locations.

GARBAGE

✔ Put garbage in a covered container.

✔ Use plastic bags for wet or greasy garbage.

✔ Dispose of regularly, *before* the container or bag is full.

FLOORS & SURFACES

✔ Wipe up spills.

✔ Use clean, soapy water or an appropriate cleaning product to clean counters and other surfaces, including the stove.

✔ Sweep floors daily.

✔ Mop floors weekly. Use clean, warm water and a detergent. Change water as it gets dirty. Do not use water on wood floors. Use a wood-floor cleaning product or a damp mop.

REFRIGERATOR

✔ Make sure refrigerator keeps food cold. If you think it may not work properly, report it to your supervisor.

✔ Regularly dispose of food that is spoiled or no longer fresh. Be sure you discuss this first with the client.

✔ Clean the inside surfaces of the refrigerator weekly.

✔ If the freezer needs to be defrosted, discuss it with your supervisor.

Bathroom

Bathrooms are used constantly and must be regularly cleaned. Wet surfaces and moisture make a good environment for germs. Wet floors are dangerous. Toilets become fouled with use. A clean bathroom is both pleasant **and safe**.

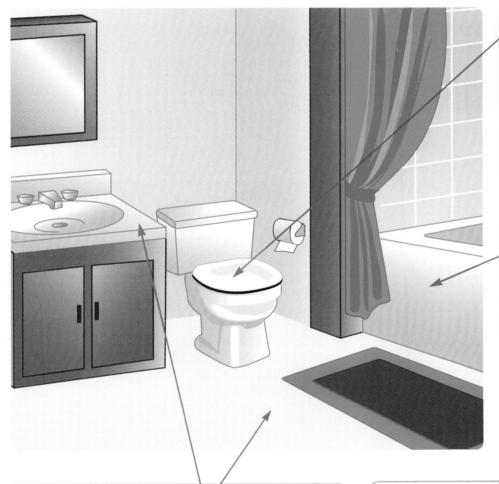

TOILETS
✔ Clean toilets weekly or as needed.

LINENS
✔ Replace towels and face cloths regularly.

TRASH
✔ Empty trash daily.

TUBS & SHOWERS
✔ Make sure bath and shower floors have non-skid surfaces.
✔ Clean tub and shower with appropriate cleanser at least every other week.

FLOORS & SURFACES
✔ Keep floors dry to prevent falls.
✔ Wipe sink daily.
✔ Open doors and windows when possible to reduce moisture.
✔ Mop floors weekly using clean, warm water and detergent.
✔ Use non-skid rugs and bath mats.

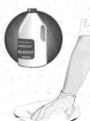

CLEANING PRODUCTS

Many cleaning products contain strong chemicals. Use rubber cleaning gloves. Keep doors and windows open if possible. **Always follow the directions on the label. Never mix different products**—some may react together to form poisonous gas. A good, basic cleaner is a solution of household bleach and water (see page 123), though it must also be handled carefully.

Laundry

Only perform laundry activities that are indicated in the care plan, activity sheet, or in other written instructions from your supervisor. If using commercial machines, make arrangements with your supervisor and the client first regarding payment.

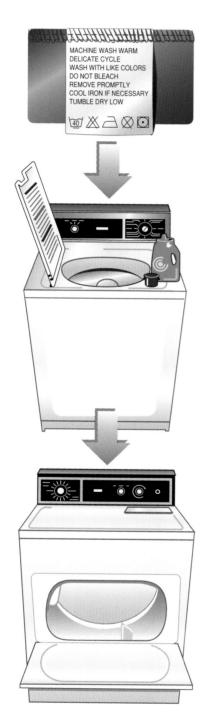

CHECK THE LABEL

It is easy to damage clothing. Most clothing has washing instructions on a label sewn into the garment. Following these instructions is important to prevent damaging the garment.

WASHING MACHINES

- Read manufacturer's directions for the machine.
- Measure and add detergent. Check washer directions and detergent label for correct amount. Add bleach if desired. Note: never pour bleach directly on clothing as it can damage or discolor garments. Dilute bleach in water.
- Sort clothing by type: colors, whites, delecates. Wash one type at a time.
- Select correct setting: normal, permanent press, delicate, etc.
- Select water temperature: hot for whites, warm or cold for colors and permanent press.
- Add liquid fabric softener if desired, following softener directions.

DRYERS

- Read manufacturer's directions for the machine and clothing labels for drying instructions.
- Sort clothing by type: normal, permanent press, etc.
- Add dryer fabric softener if desired.
- Check and clean lint filter.
- Select appropriate setting or time: normal, permanent press, etc. Don't over-dry clothing.

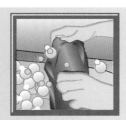

HAND-WASHING CLOTHES

You can wash clothing in a sink if the client doesn't have access to a washer.
- Wash clothing by type.
- Follow clothing label instructions.
- Be sure to rinse well.

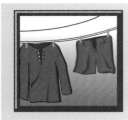

HANGING CLOTHES TO DRY

You can dry clothes on a clothes line or drying rack if the client doesn't have access to a dryer.
- Make sure the line or rack is clean.
- Make sure the clothes are secure—use clothespins on lines.
- Shake out wrinkles as you hang clothes.

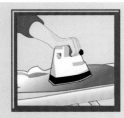

IRONING

- Follow manufacturer's instructions regarding temperature settings. Test them on clothing by using lower than indicated temperatures first and changing them as needed.
- Handle irons with care. It is easy to burn yourself or your client's clothing.
- Use an ironing board—not another flat surface like a table-top.
- Never leave on an iron unattended. It is a potential fire hazard.

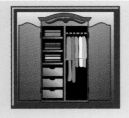

STORING CLOTHING

- Store clothing neatly. Fold neatly or hang on hangers. Poorly stored clothing will wrinkle.
- Ask clients for their preferences on storage and try to accommodate them.

Shopping & Money Management

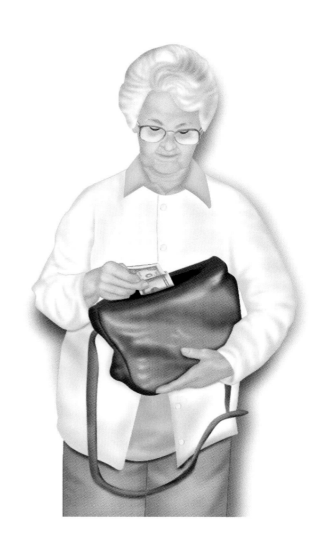

You may be required to handle clients' money.

You may have to purchase groceries and other household items for clients, or perform banking and other financial activities for them. This is a great responsibility and an area of potential conflict. It is easy to make mistakes in counting, in purchasing the wrong item, or in other ways.

Careful accounting of all money matters is necessary.

Clients may forget where their money is, or how much they have, or how much they gave you. Pay close attention to any money the client shows you or gives to you. Write down all transactions as they happen, confirm them with the client, and get receipts. Report all transactions to your agency as well. If a client is cognitively impaired, follow your supervisor's instructions for reporting to the client's guardian.

Treat clients' resources with respect.

You must spend the client's money wisely. Clients on small incomes may have to use *food stamps or discount coupons*, or shop for items on sale. All clients have to live within their resources. If you are shopping for them, shop for value and never criticize their purchase choices.

A client's financial resources are private and confidential.

Many clients may be reluctant to discuss money matters. They may be embarrassed by how little they have or fearful of having it stolen from them. Turning over money management to a stranger may also represent a loss of independence. You must not discuss a client's resources with anyone other than your supervisor and the client (or client's guardian).

Remember to follow the care plan when shopping for food.

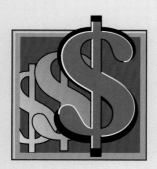

STRETCHING DOLLARS

You can save the client money when shopping by paying attention to the cost of items and by looking for discounts off normal purchase prices. Groceries can often be purchased at a discount using coupons found in local newspapers. For the cost of a newspaper, it's possible to save many times that in food expenses. It's also important to look for sales and to check the *unit price* of items. That's the price of a single unit (an ounce, for example) rather than of an entire container or package. Unit prices are often cheaper for larger quantities and may be a better buy. However, a lower unit price will not mean savings if the client will be unable to use all of the item before it spoils.

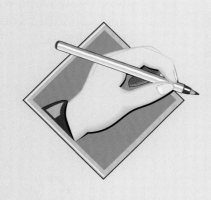

KEEPING A RECORD

It's a good idea to keep a small notebook or pad for recording transactions. Write them down as they happen because it is easy to forget. Show your notes to the client for confirmation. Your agency will have reporting requirements that you must follow. You will be expected to record:

✔ amounts received;
✔ amounts spent;
✔ amounts deposited;
✔ amounts returned.

Remember to get and keep receipts for all purchases, payments, or deposits!

Care of the Home

1.

How do you feel about having strangers in your home? What kind of behavior do you expect of them?

2.

How do you want your home to appear to guests? What do you notice about other people's homes when you visit them?

3.

What are the most important housekeeping activities to you? Why? Do you think other people feel the same way?

4.

How would you feel about giving someone else money to do your shopping? What concerns would you have about their buying what you wanted and spending your money wisely?

REVIEW

**Key Terms – Test your understanding of each of these first.
Then use each one once to fill in the incomplete statements below.**

housekeeping plan

safety

garbage

cleaning products

washing instructions

water temperature

irons

food stamps and discount coupons

unit price

receipts

1. _____ should be put in a covered container and disposed of before the container or bag is full.

2. Before washing and drying laundry, check the _____ on labels inside the clothing.

3. You will use _____ in making many purchases for clients.

4. A _____ will help you keep track of housekeeping tasks and the equipment and supplies needed to perform them.

5. Checking the _____ of items will help you get the best value when shopping for clients.

6. _____ is a fundamental goal of housekeeping.

7. _____ contain strong chemicals. Keep doors and windows open when using them.

8. When washing clothes, be sure to use the correct _____.

9. When shopping for clients, always get _____ for purchases.

10. Never leave _____ on unattended.

Safety

> **You have a responsibility to your clients, your agency, and yourself to practice safety on the job.**

As a home care aide, there will be many opportunities for accident or injury, whether you are inside the client's home or outside it. Many of these will be obvious, but some will not.

> **Awareness and communication are keys to safety.**

You can prevent accidents if you recognize *hazards* (dangerous situations likely to cause accidents). Good communication between you, your clients, and supervisor will help you prevent accidents and make accidents that occur have less serious results.

> **You will be trained in special safety techniques that you must follow.**

This course and this textbook provide guidelines for preventing infection, moving and lifting clients, handling equipment, and performing other activities safely. You will also learn how to respond to emergencies such as a choking client or a fire.

ACCIDENT PREVENTION

HOME CARE AIDE

- **Infection:** From infectious diseases (AIDS, hepatitis, etc.).
- **Lifting Injuries:** From lifting or moving clients and other heavy objects.
- **Falls:** From wet or cluttered floors, careless actions.
- **Wounds:** From knives (while preparing food) or sharp edges.
- **Assault:** From aggressive or agitated clients, or from others outside the client's home. *Note: "Street safety" is important. You must get to and from the client's home safely in order to provide care.*
- **Electrocution:** From electrical equipment.
- **Burns:** From cooking, hot liquids, cigarettes, etc.

✔ **Awareness:** Pay close attention to clients and your surroundings. Look for possible hazards.

✔ **Communication:** Report information promptly and accurately. You are your supervisor's eyes and ears.

✔ **Safety Practices:** Always keep safety in mind. Follow your agency's safety guidelines.

Hazards

CLIENT

- **Infection:** From improper infection control practices by home care providers.
- **Communication:** Any inability to communicate, whether because of cognitive impairment, medication, or a language barrier.
- **Falls:** Due to wet or cluttered floors, medication, weakness, dizziness, lack of bed rails, etc.
- **Choking:** From food, or for cognitively impaired clients from small inedible objects.
- **Poisoning:** From too much or the wrong medication
- **Burns:** From cigarettes, hot food, heat packs, hot bath, etc.
- **Suffocation:** From choking, drowning in bath, pillows, etc.

SPECIAL CLIENTS

- Normal conditions for others may be dangerous and cause accidents for the cognitively impaired. Such clients need special attention.
- Certain physical disabilities (such as paralysis) need special care to prevent serious accidents.
- Physical impairment from aging (failing eyesight, hearing, coordination, etc.) can also increase the risk of accident.
- Many disorders and conditions like decubitus ulcers, contractures, or diabetes are easily made worse through neglect or poor care.

Infection Control

Diseases are caused by microorganisms and viruses too small to be seen by the eye.

The microorganisms and viruses which cause disease are called *pathogens.* They enter the cells of the body to cause infections. When a disease is *contagious,* it can be transmitted to other people.

Contagious diseases can be spread in many ways.

Pathogens can be carried in the air as a result of sneezing or coughing. They can be spread through direct contact and through blood and body fluids to objects and to you. The skin is an excellent defense against pathogens but open cuts (which cannot always be seen by the eye) and *mucous membranes* (like those of the mouth, nose, and eyes) are easily infected.

Your contact with clients must not spread pathogens to them or to you.

Aseptic practices prevent the spread of contagious disease. They require you to have *clean conditions* (pathogen free—but not necessarily free of *harmless* microorganisms) or *sterile conditions* (free of *all* microorganisms). There are aseptic procedures for washing hands, wearing protective clothing, and disinfecting or disposing of contaminated material that will protect you and your client.

Use *Universal Precautions* to protect yourself from being infected by pathogens carried in blood and body fluids.

According to November, 1992 guidelines from the Centers for Disease Control, these safety practices apply to contact with blood, semen, vaginal secretions, and any body fluids (feces, urine, vomitus, etc.) in which you can see blood. Because you cannot always know in advance when there will be blood in a client's body fluid, **you should always use these precautions any time you will come in contact with blood and body fluids.**

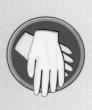

DISPOSABLE GLOVES:
- *Worn any time you will come in contact with blood and body fluids, mucous membranes, wounds, and items contaminated by them.*
- *Discarded after each client contact.*

MASKS, EYE WEAR, AND FACE SHIELDS:
- Worn when coming into contact with large or small airborne particles of blood and body fluids.

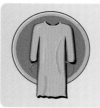

APRONS OR GOWNS:
- Worn when clothing may be contaminated by blood or body fluids.

NOTE: **If you have been exposed to blood or body fluids, you will have to file an incident or exposure report.**

HAND WASHING:

- *Before and after contact with each client.*
- Immediately if contaminated by blood or body fluid (Also wash any contaminated body areas).
- Immediately after removing gloves.

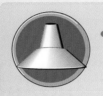

RESUSCITATION:

- Use resuscitation devices when mouth-to-mouth resuscitation is needed.

UNIVERSAL PRECAUTIONS

The Centers for Disease Control developed safety practices which are required for anyone exposed in their jobs to blood and body fluids. These practices assume all clients to be possibly infectious for HIV and other blood-borne diseases. They are based on setting up barriers to infections, decontamination of contaminated body parts and certain materials, and safe disposal of other contaminated materials.

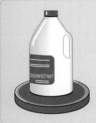

DECONTAMINATION:

- Clean up blood and body fluid spills immediately with the disinfectant recommended by your agency. Gloves must be worn for this.

SKIN LESIONS OR WEEPING DERMATITIS:

- When you have any skin wounds, lesions, or weeping dermatitis, you should stay away from direct contact with clients and client care equipment.

SHARP OBJECTS:

- Be very careful with sharp objects like razors, knives, and sharp edges of equipment to avoid cuts to yourself or to the client.

Isolation Precautions

Isolation precautions are taken with clients who have a contagious disease.

Clients with certain contagious diseases may be *isolated* in a room or area of their home. Everyone entering the isolation area must then follow isolation precautions to prevent spreading the disease. The types of isolation are listed at right.

The goal of isolation is to maintain a pathogen-proof barrier around the client.

Clean *barrier supplies* (plastic bags, gloves, masks, etc.) are kept outside the isolation area. Everything in the area is considered contaminated. Anyone leaving the area must follow the correct isolation guidelines. Contaminated linens and trash are bagged and sealed before removal. Disinfectant is used to clean all contaminated surfaces.

Isolation precautions will differ with the disease.

Universal Precautions are taken for blood and body fluid isolation. Other types of precautions are listed at right. Your supervisor and agency will inform you if you are to take isolation precautions. Follow their guidelines carefully.

Universal Precautions (p. 88-89) are the precautions used for blood and body fluid isolation. Other types of isolation precautions are:

DRAINAGE/SECRETION ISOLATION
- ✔ Gowns worn if contamination of clothing is likely.
- ✔ Gloves worn if touching wounds, drainage, or infectious material (including linens).
- ✔ Hands washed on entry and exit.
- ✔ Blood and body fluid spills are promptly cleaned with sodium hypochlorite and water solution.
- ✔ Contaminated items are put in a waste bag and labeled.

STRICT ISOLATION
- ✔ Masks.
- ✔ Gowns.
- ✔ Gloves.
- ✔ Hands washed on entry and exit.
- ✔ Contaminated items are put in a waste bag and labeled.

CONTACT ISOLATION
- ✔ Masks worn by those having direct contact with client.
- ✔ Gowns worn if contamination of clothing is likely.
- ✔ Gloves worn if infectious material will be touched.
- ✔ Hands washed on entry and exit.
- ✔ Contaminated items are put in a waste bag and labeled.

BIOHAZARD

Orange labels with these symbols indicate possibly infectious material and are put on containers for such material.

ISOLATION PRECAUTIONS

Hands are washed before entering the isolation area, after leaving, and immediately after any contamination.

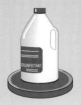

Disinfectant is used to clean all contaminated surfaces. This includes bedpans and urinals.

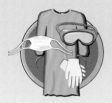

Barrier protections are used according to the type of precaution.

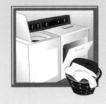

Contaminated laundry must be kept separate and washed in hot water. Handle carefully and follow your supervisor's and agency's guidelines on contaminated laundry.

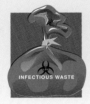

Trash, dressings, and contaminated laundry should be put in plastic bags and tightly sealed before removal from the area. Feces and urine are flushed directly down the toilet.

Dishes must be washed promptly in hot water. Dishwashers will normally disinfect contaminated dishes. If you are washing by hand, wear gloves, use hot water, and handle with care. Disinfect all surrounding surfaces when done.

RESPIRATORY ISOLATION
- ✔ Masks worn for close contact.
- ✔ Hands washed on entry and exit.
- ✔ Contaminated items are put in a waste bag and labeled.

ACID FAST BACILLUS – AFB ISOLATION
- ✔ Masks worn when client is coughing without covering mouth.
- ✔ Gowns worn by those having direct contact with client.
- ✔ Hands washed on entry and exit.
- ✔ Contaminated items are put in a waste bag and labeled.

ENTERIC (INTESTINAL) ISOLATION
- ✔ Masks worn by those having direct contact with client.
- ✔ Gowns worn if contamination of clothing is likely.
- ✔ Gloves worn if client or infectious material (including linens) will be touched.
- ✔ Hands washed on entry and exit.
- ✔ Contaminated items are put in a waste bag and labeled.

Body Mechanics

Home care aides lift and move clients, supplies, and equipment every day.

If not performed correctly, these activities can result in serious injury or damage. You may hurt a client, co-worker, or yourself or damage property.

You must follow basic principles of fitness and body mechanics to properly perform these activities.

You will need strength and flexibility in back, abdominal, arm, and leg muscles. Regular exercise and stretching of these muscles will prepare you. Practicing good body mechanics will help you avoid injury.

You will also learn specific techniques for lifting, moving, or repositioning clients.

The human body is a flexible object. When lifted or moved, it reacts differently than a fixed object like a box. Client behavior and condition will also affect movement. It will be important for you to know how clients will react as you help move them.

✔ USE YOUR LEG MUSCLES

Your back is easily injured. **Bend your knees, not your back.** This will put pressure on the powerful leg muscles which can better absorb it.

Always keep your back straight.

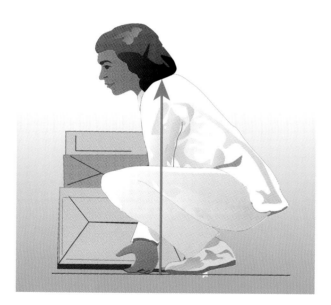

OTHER DO'S
- ✔ Stay fit. Stay flexible.
- ✔ Push, pull, or roll objects rather than lifting them whenever you can.
- ✔ Decide if you need help and get it when you do.

Lower back injuries are the leading cause of work-related injuries for home care aides.

✔ KEEP OBJECTS CLOSE TO YOUR BODY

The closer the object's weight is to your own **center of gravity** (between your hips) the easier it will be to maintain balance and transfer pressure to leg muscles.

Leaning or reaching will strain back and other muscles.

✔ KEEP HIPS AND SHOULDERS SQUARED

Face the object with hips and shoulders squared, whether lifting, pushing, or pulling. **When you turn, pivot your feet instead of twisting at the waist.** This will help you keep your balance and distribute the pressure of the object evenly.

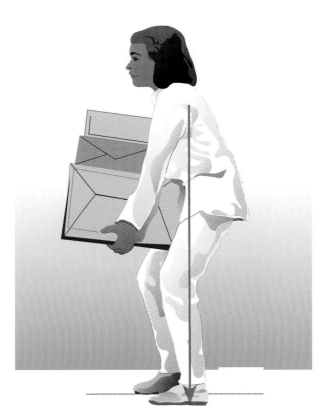

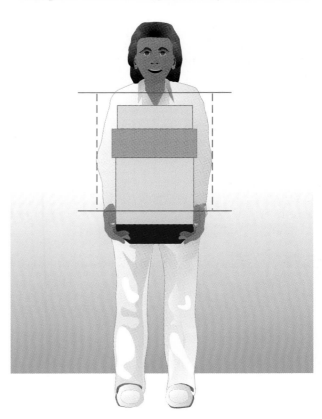

DON'TS

✘ Twist your upper body.
✘ Bend your back.
✘ Strain—the object is too heavy.
✘ Jerk at objects or make sudden moves.

✘ Try anything you are not sure you can handle —get help.
✘ Lift heavy objects when feeling weak or dizzy.

Fire & Disaster Preparedness

Fires and other disasters (like floods or blizzards) can require you to evacuate a client's home. Safe practices, careful planning, and knowledge of emergency procedures can save lives, including your own.

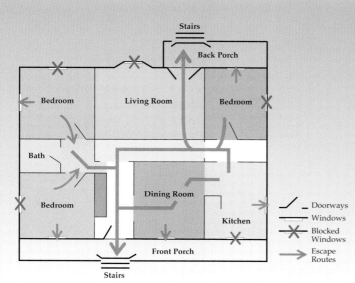

Evacuation Plan

The **first** thing you should do on entering the client's home for the first time is prepare an evacuation plan.

✔ Draw a rough plan of the home and note doors and windows that can be used for escape.

✔ Check the doors and windows to see that they can be opened easily. Make sure you know how to open any special locks or burglar barriers quickly.

✔ Plan where you will go once outside the home.

✔ Discuss your escape plan with the client and the client's family so they will know what to do.

Fire Prevention

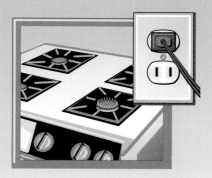

Most fires are preventable. Common causes of fire include carelessness with open flames while cooking or smoking and the misuse of electrical cords and equipment. Follow these guidelines and your agency's policy of fire prevention:

✔ **Never leave cooking unattended.**

✔ When using gas stoves, keep clothing and other inflammable objects away from flames.

✔ Make sure pilot lights for gas stoves, heaters, and water heaters are working. Report gas odors to the utility company immediately and be prepared to evacuate everyone from the home.

✔ Cigarette smoking should be done carefully and **never in bed.**

✔ **Plug appliances directly into wall outlets, not extension cords or adapters.**

✔ Worn electrical cords or malfunctioning equipment should not be used.

✔ **Check smoke detectors** frequently to make sure they work.

✔ Where *oxygen therapy* is used, no smoking is allowed, electrical appliances should not be used, inflammable liquids are removed, and static-causing fabrics like wool and synthetics are prohibited. Only cotton uniforms, linens, etc. are allowed.

✔ Know where extinguishers are and read the instructions on how to use them **before** there is a fire.

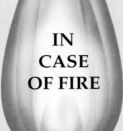

evacuate: to remove people from danger to safety.
inflammable: easy to set on fire.

IN CASE OF FIRE

Evacuate

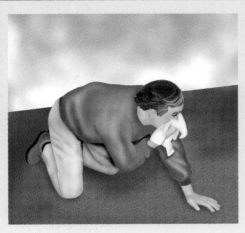

✔ **Calmly remove clients and anyone needing assistance from the home to a safe location.**
✔ **Smoke kills. Bend or crawl beneath it. Do not breathe it.** If there is a large amount of smoke, cover your mouth and your client's with a handkerchief or other cloth.
✔ **Do not use elevators.** You could be trapped in one if electrical power shuts off. Elevator shafts spread smoke and fire.
✔ **If possible, close doors and windows behind you.** This will slow the spread of the fire because it limits the oxygen the fire needs.

Alarm

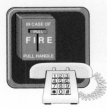

As soon as you are certain everyone is safe, call for help. Depending on the situation, you may call the fire department, activate a fire alarm, or alert some other person like a building superintendent or neighbor. You should note the location of the fire, its size, and any information (such as possible hazards) that you think might help firefighters. **Quick communication may save lives and property.**

Stop, Drop, Roll

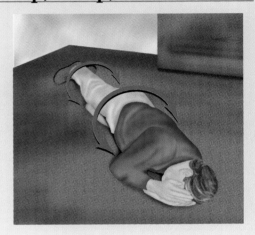

If your clothes or someone else's catch fire, it can be put out by doing the following:

✔ **Stop** immediately. Running will increase the fire.
✔ **Drop** to the ground and cover your face with your hands.
✔ **Roll** over on the floor until the fire is out.

Extinguish

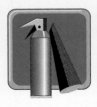

Fighting fires is a dangerous job best left to professionals. However, you may be able to put out small fires (like one in a frying pan or a wastebasket). Baking soda can be sprinkled on a pan fire to put it out. Keep it handy when cooking. You should also know where there is a fire extinguisher and how to use it if necessary. You then need to use good judgment in deciding whether to try to put out the fire. **If you have any doubt about your ability to put out a small fire quickly, evacuate the home and call for help.**

Safety

1.

Everyone has accidents. Make a list of five accidents (small or large) which you have had recently. Why did they happen? What can you do differently to prevent them happening again.

2.

Make a list of all the potential hazards a home care aide might find in your home.

3.

Prepare a fire drill for your apartment or home by imagining that an electrical fire occurs in your bedroom wall one night. Write down the steps you would take. Compare this to the guidelines on pages 94-95.

4.

Imagine that you are a client who cannot get out of bed and that there is a fire in your home. How do you think you would feel? What would you want the home care aide helping you to do?

REVIEW

**Key Terms – Test your understanding of each of these first.
Then use each one once to fill in the incomplete statements below.**

infection, lifting injuries, & falls

pathogens

mucous membranes

aseptic

sterile

universal precautions

isolation precautions

biohazard

body mechanics

fire prevention

evacuation plan

oxygen therapy

1. The_____ symbol indicates containers for potentially infectious material.

2. Disease-causing microorganisms are called _____.

3. When _____ is used, no smoking is allowed.

4. Good _____ while lifting, pushing, or pulling means keeping your back straight, staying balanced, and using your leg muscles.

5. _____ requires awareness of potential hazards (such as lit cigarettes or worn electrical cords).

6. _____ are common hazards for home care aides.

7. The first thing you should do upon entering a client's home for the first time is prepare an _____ .

8. _____ practice is pathogen free. If an object is _____, it is free of all microorganisms.

9. Open cuts and any of the body's _____ are easily penetrated by pathogens.

10. When _____ are ordered, a barrier is created to prevent the spread of pathogens. _____ create a barrier against blood-borne pathogens.

Client Emergencies

Sometimes, an unexpected and severe problem endangers a client.

Choking, unconsciousness, falling injuries, and wounds are among the many emergencies that can happen to clients. The basic practices for responding to emergencies are outlined in this unit. Preparation, quick assessment and action, and good communication are necessary for handling emergencies successfully. A client's life can depend on how you react to such situations.

Your agency will have policies about how to handle emergency situations.

They will tell you what you can and cannot do, and when and how to get assistance. You must be completely familiar with these policies and always ready to follow them. They may also require you to take special training in *cardiopulmonary resuscitation (CPR),* a rescue procedure for people whose heartbeat and breathing have stopped.

Remain calm in an emergency.

You will need to think clearly and act quickly and confidently. If you lose control of your actions, you will not be effective. Being prepared for emergencies will help you react better when they actually happen. Learn the steps on these pages and your agency's policies—and always use safe practices so you encounter as few emergencies as possible.

1. ASSESS THE SITUATION

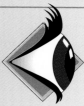

- ✔ Try to quickly **determine the cause of the problem.** This may help in treating the victim. It will also help **avoid placing yourself in any danger.** For example, if the victim has fallen because the floor is slippery, you may fall too unless you proceed carefully. You will be of no help to the victim if you become injured.

- ✔ **Notice the time.** This can be especially important if the victim loses consciousness.

4. DO NO HARM

- ✔ While you wait for assistance, **make victims as comfortable as possible without moving them.** Moving an accident victim can aggravate an injury.

- ✔ **Never perform life-saving procedures on victims unless you are sure they are necessary.** Unnecessary procedures can cause injury.

- ✔ **Never try a procedure you are not trained and authorized to perform.**

2. ASSESS THE VICTIM

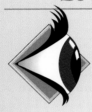

✔ Ask the victim what has happened and if he or she is injured. The victim's response or lack of response will tell you **if he or she is conscious and able to communicate.**

✔ If the victim responds, **do not accept what he or she says as the exact truth.** For example, a victim of a fall may be too embarrassed to tell you of a serious injury.

✔ **Check for visible signs of injury.** Check for breathing and pulse if the victim appears to be unconscious.

3. GET ASSISTANCE

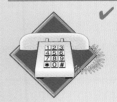

✔ Most emergencies will require you to **immediately call a nurse, emergency medical service personnel (EMS), or a physician.** Follow your agency policy. Be sure you know who to call **before** an emergency occurs.

5. PROVIDE EMOTIONAL SUPPORT

✔ The emergency victim will often show signs of the stress he or she is experiencing (fear, anger, etc.). A calm and confident manner on your part will reassure the victim. **Listen carefully to what the victim tells you and inform him or her of the actions you are taking.**

6. REPORT THE INCIDENT

✔ You will have to file an **incident report.** Learn your agency's reporting guidelines on emergencies and be prepared to correctly report any incidents. Remember that **the information you observe may be of direct value to the treatment of the victim.**

The Heimlich Maneuver

Choking on food is a common problem that can be fatal.

When food is stuck in the throat, it blocks the flow of air to the lungs. If the blockage is complete, the victim will die unless the food is quickly removed.

Grabbing the throat is a natural reaction to choking.

If you see someone grabbing his or her throat, notice quickly if the person is able to cough. **If the person is able to cough, speak, or breathe, let him or her cough out the food:** the person's airway is not completely blocked. **If the person is not able to cough, speak, or breathe, you should perform the Heimlich Maneuver immediately:** the airway is completely blocked and the person will die unless the blockage is removed.

The Heimlich Maneuver forces food blockages out of the airway.

A series of thrusts to the abdomen (stomach) forces air out of the lungs and into the airway. The pressure of these bursts of air can force food blockages out of the airway and allow normal breathing to resume. You should always be ready to use the Heimlich Maneuver. You can save someone's life.

PROCEDURE

1. ASSESS AND RESPOND

- Check that the victim is choking. **If the victim can speak or cough, leave him or her alone.** If not, stand behind the victim.
- Put your arms around the victim's waist, making a fist with one hand.

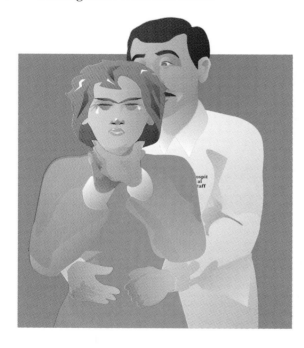

➡ *Remember to follow the guidelines for client emergencies on page 98-99.*

POINTERS

2. POSITION HANDS

- Place your fist with the thumb side against the abdomen midway between the waist and rib cage.
- Grasp your fist with the other hand.

3. THRUST

- Pull your fist with your other hand inward and upward into the center of the abdomen in a smooth, quick motion.
- Repeat four times.

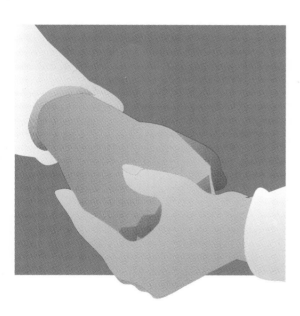

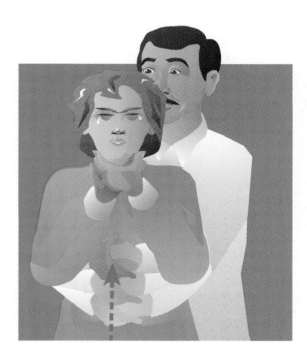

➡ *Make sure your fist is thrusting into the center of the victim's abdomen. Do not squeeze with your arms.*

➡ *If the airway remains blocked and the victim loses consciousness, perform a finger sweep (see page 103).*

➡ *The Heimlich Maneuver may not work with obese victims and should not be used with infants or clearly pregnant women.*

The Heimlich Maneuver On A Supine Victim

If a choking victim loses consciousness or is otherwise unable to stand, the Heimlich Maneuver can be performed with the victim positioned on his or her back (the *supine* position).

PROCEDURE

1. STRADDLE VICTIM

- Sit across (straddle) the victim's thighs.
- Place the heel of one hand on the abdomen between the waist and the rib cage.

2. THRUST

- Place the other hand over the first hand and **push the heel of that hand inward and upward into the victim's abdomen.** Repeat four times.

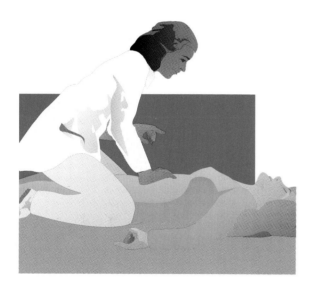

➥ *You may find it easier to straddle one thigh.*

➥ *Notice the time the victim loses consciousness. Emergency personnel may need to know this.*

➥ **Be careful not to push on the rib cage.**

➥ *Perform a finger sweep (page 103) if the victim loses consciousness.*

POINTERS

The Finger Sweep

If the Heimlich Maneuver has not cleared a blocked airway and the victim loses consciousness, try to clear the airway with the finger sweep. **Because of the risk of infection, you will need to wear disposable gloves.**

1. JAW LIFT

- Wearing gloves, grasp the victim's tongue and lower jaw by placing the thumb of the hand closest to the victim's chest into his or her mouth and over the tongue.
- Place the other fingers over the jaw and lift.

2. FINGER SWEEP

- With the index finger of your other hand, feel around the base of the tongue for any foreign objects. **Using your finger as a hook, carefully sweep any objects up into the mouth and remove them.**

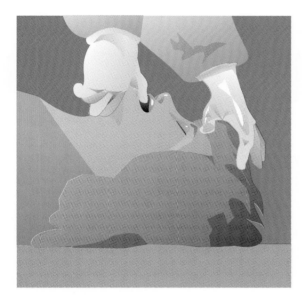

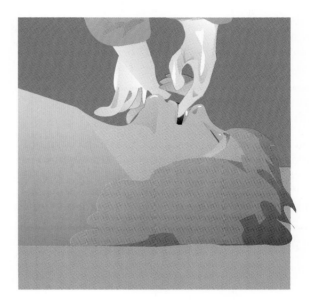

➡ *Be careful not to push the object further into the airway.*

➡ *If the airway remains blocked after performing the Heimlich Maneuver and the finger sweep, you will need to get emergency assistance immediately.*

➡ *Remember to follow the guidelines for client emergencies on page 98-99.*

Unconscious Victim

Always check the airway, breathing, and circulation (A-B-C) of the unconscious victim.

This will tell you if unconsciousness is due to the failure of the lungs to breathe air (respiratory arrest) or the heart to pump blood (cardiac arrest). If either is true, death will follow quickly unless *cardiopulmonary resuscitation (CPR)* or other life-saving efforts are applied.

CPR can only be applied by someone formally trained in the procedure.

CPR is a rescue procedure for people whose heartbeat and breathing have stopped. In CPR, you blow air into the victim's mouth and push on the victim's chest over the heart. This puts air in the lungs and keeps blood flowing through the heart.

Your agency may require you to have CPR training.

If you are not trained in CPR, you will have to notify someone who is, such as a nurse or emergency medical service worker (EMS), when CPR is needed. You will then tell them the information you have learned from your ABC assessment of the victim.

Be prepared to act quickly.

Always notice the time. You only have minutes to restore breathing or circulation before the victim is seriously hurt. **If you are not trained in CPR, know how to get assistance and do so immediately.** Remember to follow the client emergency guidelines on pages 98-99.

A. AIRWAY

- **If you are sure there is no neck or spinal injury, open the airway by performing a head-tilt.**
- While kneeling next to the victim, place the fingers of one hand under the edge of the victim's chin and of the other hand on the forehead.
- Gently lift the chin and tilt the head back so that the mouth and airway are open.

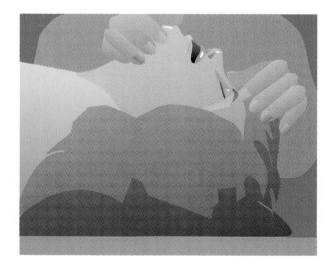

➡ *Never move an unconscious person unless he or she is in a dangerous area and it is absolutely necessary. If it is, be sure to carefully support the neck and spine.*

POINTERS

B. BREATHING

- With the head tilted back, place your ear near the victim's mouth and nose.
- **Look** at the victim's chest to see if it is rising and falling.
- **Listen** for the sound of breathing.
- **Feel** for warm air being exhaled from the victim's mouth and nose.

C. CIRCULATION

- Stabilize the head in the tilted position with the hand on the forehead.
- **Place the tips of the index and middle fingers of the other hand on the hollow of the neck closest to you.**
- Check the **carotid artery** for a pulse.

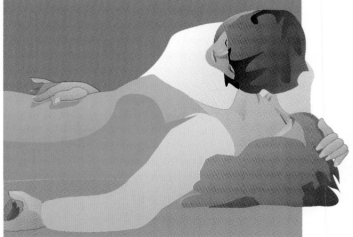

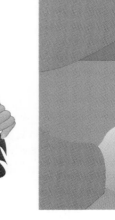

➡ *If there is no pulse, the victim has suffered cardiac arrest. CPR must be performed as soon as possible.*

➡ *See pages 60, 246, and 247 for more on checking the pulse.*

➡ *If the victim is not breathing, he or she has suffered respiratory arrest.*

Fallen Client

Falls are common accidents for the ill and the elderly. They can result in serious injury, including flesh wounds, broken bones, and damage to internal organs. Your agency will have a policy on how you should respond to a fall and how you must report the incident.

ASSESS THE SITUATION

- Has the victim fallen because the floor is slippery or cluttered? If so, **act in a safe way that will not result in your falling.**

ASSESS THE VICTIM

- Find out what happened and if there are any signs of bleeding or broken bones (sharp pain, discoloration, deformity, swelling). **Check life-threatening problems first** (unconsciousness, respiratory arrest, cardiac arrest, severe bleeding).

GET ASSISTANCE

- Follow agency policy on whom to call.

DO NO HARM

- **If there are any broken bones, do not attempt to move or reposition the victim unless he or she is in a life-threatening position.** Fractures may be painful and disturbing but are generally not life-threatening. However, there may be a more serious injury to organs, nerves, or blood vessels that will be aggravated by movement.

- **If you must move or reposition the victim, carefully support the neck and spine. If you move the victim, stop at the first sign of increased pain.**

- If there is bleeding, attempt to control it according to the hemorrhage guidelines on the next page.

PROVIDE EMOTIONAL SUPPORT

- The victim may be under severe stress or simply embarrassed. Either way, a calm and supportive manner will reassure him or her.

REPORT THE INCIDENT.

- Follow agency policy.

Hemorrhages

A hemorrhage is excessive bleeding from external wounds or internal injury. Internal hemorrhaging may be seen in skin discoloration or blood in the urine, feces, or vomitus. Hemorrhage victims may go into shock (falling blood pressure, weak pulse, and confusion caused by blood loss), lose consciousness, and die if the hemorrhaging is not stopped.

ASSESS THE SITUATION

- **Remember to use Universal Precautions (pages 88-89) anytime you come into contact with blood.** You should always have an extra pair of latex gloves for this possibility.

ASSESS THE VICTIM

- Find out what happened. See if the hemorrhaging is the most severe problem and check for consciousness, respiratory arrest, or cardiac arrest.

GET ASSISTANCE

- Follow agency policy on whom to call.

DO NO HARM

- **While you are waiting for assistance, apply direct pressure to wounds with a sterile gauze pad.** This may help the wound to clot.
- **If the wound does not stop after five minutes, apply pressure to the major artery that supplies blood to the wound area** by pressing your middle three fingers over the arterial pressure point (see page 60-61). Do not cut off all circulation.

PROVIDE EMOTIONAL SUPPORT

- The victim may be confused and under severe stress. Either way, a calm and supportive manner will reassure him or her.

REPORT THE INCIDENT.

- Follow agency policy.

Seizures

Seizures are uncontrollable temporary disorders with symptoms of fainting, loss of consciousness, and muscle spasms. They can have many causes, including fever, changes in blood sugar, head trauma, and epilepsy. They may be major incidents requiring immediate medical attention or be barely noticeable and last only seconds.

ASSESS THE SITUATION

- If the victim is unconscious because of a seizure, the muscles will be rigid and will soon have spasms. Be prepared.

ASSESS THE VICTIM

- Is the victim having a major seizure? Has the victim injured his or her head in a fall? Does the victim have a high fever? Is he or she diabetic or epileptic?

GET ASSISTANCE

- Follow agency policy on whom to call.

DO NO HARM

- **If the victim is in a chair, gently lower him or her to the floor.**

- Place a pillow or rolled towel under the victim's head and turn the head to the side. Loosen clothing. **Cushion the victim and any nearby immovable objects as much as possible. Clear the immediate area of any objects the victim may hit.**

- **Never attempt to restrain the victim.** After spasms are finished, position the victim on his or her side.

PROVIDE EMOTIONAL SUPPORT

- The victim may be confused and embarrassed. Stay with the victim and reassure him or her as much as possible.

REPORT THE INCIDENT.

- Follow agency policy.

Stroke

A stroke (cerebrovascular accident) is an interruption of blood flow to the brain from a blockage or a hemorrhage. It damages or kills brain tissue. Symptoms include seizures, unconsciousness, paralysis, difficult breathing, hard to understand or no speech, and blurred vision.

ASSESS THE SITUATION

- A stroke victim will not endanger you, but you should still be alert to any hazards that might interfere with your ability to aid the victim.

ASSESS THE VICTIM

- Can the victim communicate? Has he or she lost consciousness? Is the victim experiencing stiffness or paralysis anywhere? **Is the victim clearly affected on one side of the body?** How are the victim's breathing and pulse?

GET ASSISTANCE

- Follow agency policy on whom to call.

DO NO HARM

- **The victim should be gently placed on his or her back, with the head slightly elevated.** This will reduce pressure to the brain.

PROVIDE EMOTIONAL SUPPORT

- The victim may be very frightened and confused, especially if they are experiencing paralysis, loss of speech **(aphasia)**, or difficult breathing. Stay with the victim and reassure him or her as much as possible. **If the victim has aphasia, he or she can still understand what you are saying.**

REPORT THE INCIDENT.

- Follow agency policy.

Poisoning

Poisoning may occur from ingesting medications, household chemicals, or spoiled food. It can also occur from breathing poisonous gases or from insect bites. Symptoms include stomach cramps, pain, nausea, vomiting, convulsions and unconsciousness. When poisoning occurs, you must determine the source of the poison and get help quickly.

ASSESS THE SITUATION

- Is there any obvious source? Do you notice any unusual odor? Note that Carbon Monoxide from faulty heating equipment has no odor.

ASSESS THE VICTIM

- Is the victim breathing and conscious? If so, ask the victim to tell you his or her symptoms. If the victim is unconscious, inspect the victim's mouth and smell his or her breath for signs of poison.

GET ASSISTANCE

- **If you suspect poisoning, get help immediately.** Follow agency policy on whom to call. There are *poison control centers* in most areas and you may be directed to call one.

DO NO HARM

- **If you suspect gas poisoning,** open windows immediately. If the problem is gas from the oven, turn it off. Assist the victim out of the area to get fresh air.

- **If you suspect chemical poisoning, do not induce vomiting.** You may be directed to give the victim water or milk to dilute the poison. If there is vomitus, save some for analysis.

PROVIDE EMOTIONAL SUPPORT

- The victim may be confused and embarrassed. Stay with the victim and reassure him or her as much as possible.

REPORT THE INCIDENT.

- Follow agency policy.

Burns

Burns from cooking and hot liquids (including bath water) are common problems in the home. Burns are painful but small ones are rarely serious. Severe burns, however, can be be very serious and even life threatening. Note that burns can have a more serious effect on children because of their small size. Review the discussion of burns on page 51.

ASSESS THE SITUATION

● Is the victim in further danger? If clothing is on fire, see directions on page 95. If the burn is from a hot surface, such as a pan, don't touch the surface yourself.

ASSESS THE VICTIM

● Is the burn minor or major? Is the skin red, swollen, blistered, or broken?

GET ASSISTANCE

● Follow agency policy on whom to call.

DO NO HARM

● **Never apply pressure to burn areas.**

● **If the burn is minor, apply a cold, wet compress or put the burn area in cold water.**

● **If the burn is severe, lightly cover with a sterile cloth.**

PROVIDE EMOTIONAL SUPPORT

● The victim will experience intense pain and may go into shock. He or she may be confused and embarrassed. Stay with the victim and reassure him or her as much as possible.

REPORT THE INCIDENT.

● Follow agency policy.

Client Emergencies

1.
Think of an emergency (sudden accident, injury, illness, etc.) you have personally experienced. How did you react?

2.
If you were an emergency victim, how would you want a home care aide to respond to your emergency?

3.
Make a list of who to contact in case of an emergency at your home. List their phone numbers, when to contact them, and what information should be provided. What general rules about getting assistance have you used in collecting this information?

4.
Imagine one of the emergencies discussed in this unit occurs. Do you feel ready to successfully respond to it? Why or why not?

REVIEW

**Key Terms – Test your understanding of each of these first.
Then use each one once to fill in the incomplete statements below.**

assessment

do no harm

choking

heimlich maneuver

finger sweep

ABC

fractures

hemorrhages

seizures

stroke

poisoning

burns

1. _____ stands for airway, breathing, and circulation—the first steps in the care of an unconscious victim.

2. Bone _____, though painful and disturbing, are not usually life-threatening.

3. Never apply pressure to _____.

4. _____ are temporary uncontrollable disorders with symptoms of fainting, loss of consciousness, and muscle spasms.

5. When _____ is suspected, it is critical that you try to determine the source.

6. The airway of a _____ victim is obstructed, and can often be cleared by applying the _____.

7. _____ from open wounds can sometimes be stopped by applying direct pressure with a sterile gauze pad.

8. The symptoms of a _____ (aphasia, unconsciousness, paralysis, etc.) can be especially frightening to the victim.

9. If a client is unconscious due to an obstructed airway, and the Heimlich maneuver has not succeeded, you may try a _____.

10. _____ of the situation and the victim is your first step in an emergency.

11. When responding to emergencies, a fundamental rule is to _____.

Preparation

*There are routine practices you must follow to begin nursing care. These practices are represented throughout this book by the **Preparation Symbol**. We have chosen a circle to emphasize that these practices work together as a system for providing basic care. Use the information on these pages and the infection control procedures that follow as your guide. You should memorize this information. When you see the **Preparation Symbol**, you will be required to use it.*

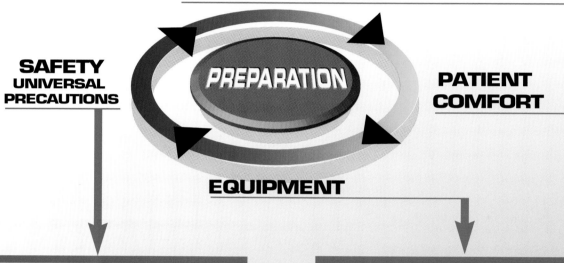

COMMUNICATION

SAFETY
UNIVERSAL PRECAUTIONS

PREPARATION

PATIENT COMFORT

EQUIPMENT

Be sensitive to possible hazards to you and the client: contaminated surfaces, conditions that could cause falls, etc.

✔ **Wash your hands before every procedure and as indicated by the presentation on the next pages.**

✔ **Follow the Universal Precautions on pages 88-89 anytime you expect to come in contact with a client's body fluids.**

✔ If the client has a hospital-type bed, position it at a comfortable height for you to work.

✔ Position the client safely. When in bed, the client should be in the center of the bed, not near the edge. Use side rails when appropriate.

✔ Use good body mechanics when lifting (pages 92-93).

✔ Get assistance in advance whenever you think there's a chance you will need it. Sometimes, (especially for confused clients) this means having someone to witness your actions.

Make sure you know the equipment or materials you need and how to use them.

✔ Make sure you bring, or have in the client's home, all the supplies you will need.

✔ Before beginning a procedure, collect all the supplies and equipment you need to complete it. **Never stop a procedure to get material or equipment.**

✔ Check to see if anything is broken, contaminated, or otherwise not able to be used.

✔ Put everything in an order that will make use easier.

✔ Bring a black ink pen and any forms or note paper you need to record results.

✔ Always have an extra pair of latex gloves.

✔ Make sure you know and follow your agency's policy on buying and being reimbursed for supplies.

Always maintain the client's right to privacy, dignity, and physical comfort.

✔ Always knock on closed doors before entering the client's room.

✔ Allow the client time to prepare for the procedure.

✔ When you're ready to begin, ask any visitors to leave.

✔ Close the client's door if there are other people in the home.

✔ Position the client so he or she is as comfortable as possible.

✔ Adjust lighting and temperature to make the client comfortable.

✔ Be sensitive to odors that might offend the client (from waste, disinfectants, your own body, etc.) and correct the situation.

✔ Only expose the parts of the client's body necessary to the procedure.

✔ Make sure clients are covered comfortably when moving them.

Be clear, accurate, and observant. Pay attention to the client's feelings.

✔ Announce your entrance with a knock and a greeting *(Hello, Good morning, etc.).*

✔ Call the client the name he or she wishes to be called.

✔ Explain the procedure in terms the client will understand. Be sensitive to any hearing or language difficulties. Let the client know when he or she can help.

✔ Ask the client if he or she understands and is ready.

✔ Write down observations as soon as possible.

✔ Report problems according to agency policy.

✔ Pay attention to what clients tell you.

✔ Do not criticize or debate clients. Accept their opinions.

Handwashing

Handwashing is your best defense against spreading infection.

Infectious germs can live on the skin for different lengths of time. Vigorous handwashing, properly performed, washes off microorganisms and protects you from infecting yourself or others.

PROCEDURE

1. PREPARATION

- Roll up sleeves. Remove watch or push it up your forearm. Turn on faucets. Use warm water.

- If you are using a bar of soap, rinse it first and hold it throughout lathering. If using a dispenser, apply liquid soap.

- Wet your wrists and then your hands, keeping both below elbow level, angled to let water run down into the sink.

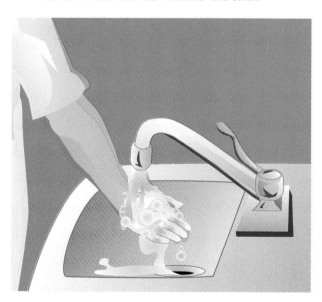

➡ *Check to see that soap and paper towels are ready for use and that there is a wastebasket before you begin.*

➡ **Stand back from the sink to prevent contact with your clothes.**

2. LATHER AND RUB

- Lather up all areas, including between fingers and backs of wrists and hands.

- Vigorously rub all areas for about 60 seconds.

- Clean your nails by rubbing them into the palm of your other hand.

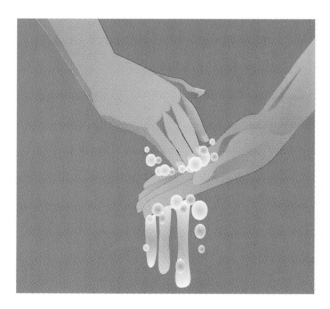

➡ *Be sure to use enough soap to get a thick lather. It loosens the microorganisms so they can be washed away by water.*

➡ *Orange sticks, brushes, or a clean damp paper towel can also be used to clean nails.*

POINTERS

WHEN TO WASH

- When you enter the client's home.
- Before and after every procedure.
- Before and after wearing gloves.
- Before preparing food.
- Before handling any items to be given to clients (meal tray, medicine, etc.).
- After handling any items used by clients (meal tray, clothing, etc.).
- Anytime your hands (or any other body parts) are contaminated with blood or body fluids.
- Anytime you use the bathroom.
- Whenever you are in doubt.

---

3. RINSE

- Rinse thoroughly, **making sure water runs down from the wrists to the fingertips.**

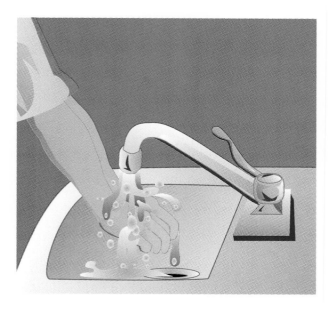

➡ *The sink is a contaminated surface. If your hands touch it at any time, start over.*

4. COMPLETE

- **Dry with a clean paper towel.** Discard towel.
- **Turn off faucet with a clean and dry paper towel.** Discard towel.
- Use skin lotion if frequent washing irritates your skin. Chapped skin is more easily infected.

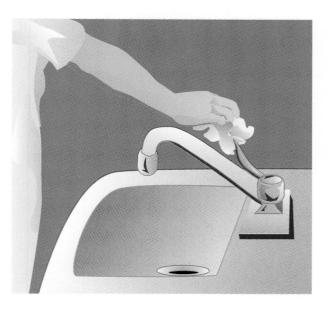

➡ *Never cut corners. Handwashing is the most important step in infection control.*

➡ *You should not wear rings or bracelets while working because of the difficulty of keeping them (and your hands) clean.*

Gowns, Aprons, Masks

You must wear protective barriers when isolation precautions (pages 90-91) are ordered. Disposable *gowns* or *aprons* are a barrier against contamination of your body or clothing by blood or body fluids. Gowns have sleeves with tight cuffs. Aprons have no sleeves but protect chest and leg areas. Disposable *face masks* are used to protect your respiratory tract.

They are always thrown away after each use.

GOWNS
PROCEDURE

1. PREPARATION	**2. FASTEN TIES**
• Take off watches and jewelry. • Roll sleeves above elbow. • Wash hands. • Unfold gown and put arms into sleeves.	• Fasten velcro tie behind neck. If using strings, tie in a bow knot. • Overlap the edges of the gown behind you so that the gown covers clothes completely. • Fasten waist-level velcro tie behind back. If using string, tie in a bow knot.

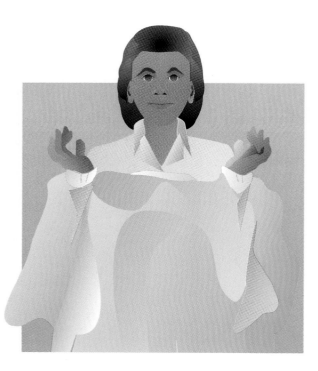

➥ *The guidelines for using an apron are basically the same as for a gown. An apron has a neck loop that slips over the head. When removing, treat it like a gown and roll inside out.*

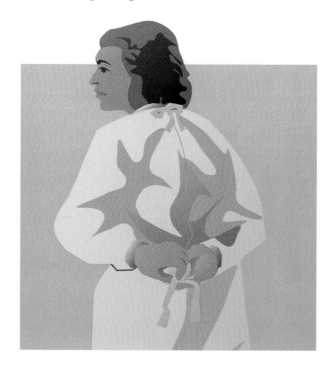

➥ *When using strings, make sure your knots will not come loose accidentally yet can be untied easily.*

POINTERS

PROTECTIVE BARRIERS

- When using protective barriers, you'll put them on in this order:

  1. gown or apron
  2. mask
  3. gloves

- You must wash your hands once in the beginning and then again after you have removed the barriers which come off in reverse order:

  1. gloves
  2. mask
  3. gown or apron

MASKS

3. REMOVAL

- When finished, remove the gown by untying the strings at the neck and waist.

- Using the strings, pull the gown away from your shoulders, turning inside out.

- Roll the gown into a ball, touching only the inside. Discard into designated container.

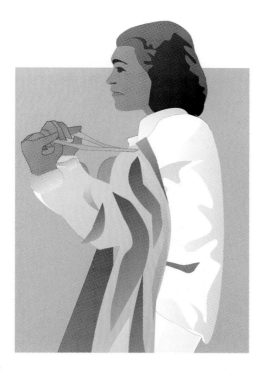

➡ *You'll remove your gloves and mask (if worn) before you remove your gown or apron.*

APPLICATION AND REMOVAL

- Position the mask over nose and mouth by holding the elastic or strings, not the mask.

- Pull elastic or tie strings above ears so that the mask is secure.

- Remove by pulling elastic over head or untying strings. Don't touch the mask itself. Discard.

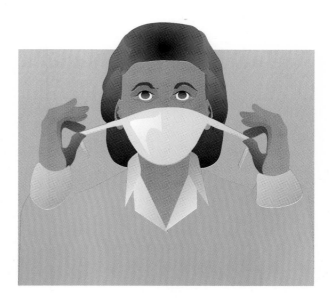

➡ *Cup masks slip on with elastic and have a clip to fit against the nose.*

➡ *Masks, gowns, aprons, and gloves can be frightening to clients. Explain that you are required to wear them as a precaution and be sensitive to the client's concerns.*

Gloves

Disposable gloves provide a two-way barrier for the hands against pathogens. They are easy to use, though you may have to get used to using them with small objects. Once contaminated, they must be handled carefully to prevent contamination of the hands or other areas.

They are always thrown away after each use.

PROCEDURE

1. WEARING GLOVES

- **Wash hands. Check gloves for tears.**
- Put gloves on so that they fit smoothly and are not too big or loose.
- When wearing a gown, gloves are pulled over the cuffs of the gown.

2. REMOVE FIRST GLOVE

- To remove, pinch one glove below the cuff. Be careful not to touch your gown or wrist.
- Pull the glove so that it turns inside out as you remove it.
- Discard into a basket or bag for contaminated trash or place into the palm of your gloved hand.

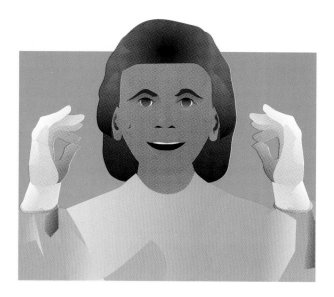

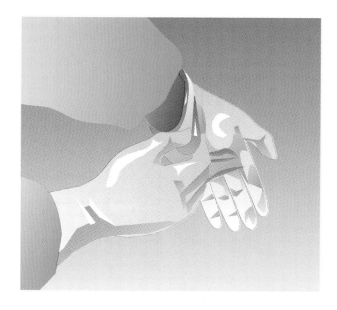

➥ *Disposable gloves tear easily. Remove rings with sharp edges.*

➥ *Always carry an extra set.*

➥ *Don't touch outside of gloves with bare hand.*

POINTERS

3. REMOVE SECOND GLOVE

- Put finger of ungloved hand inside cuff of remaining glove.
- Push down so that cuff turns inside out but hand remains gloved.

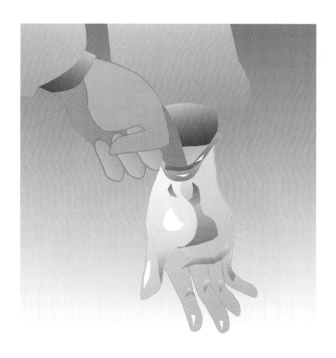

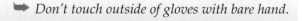
➡ *Don't touch outside of gloves with bare hand.*

4. DISCARD AND COMPLETE

- Grasp **inside of cuff** and remove glove so that it comes off inside out.
- Discard into a designated container. (If wearing gown and mask, remove them next following guidelines on pages 118-119)
- **Wash hands.**

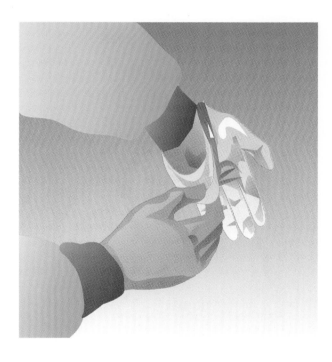

➡ *Don't touch outside of gloves with bare hand.*

Contaminated Material

Whenever you are exposed to body fluids or when Isolation Precautions are indicated, you will handle materials that could be infectious. You will seal these materials in plastic bags in the client's room before removing them. You will also clean contaminated areas in the client's room to prevent further contamination. Learn your agency's policies and procedures on handling contaminated material and follow the guidelines on these pages.

HANDLE CAREFULLY

- The BIOHAZARD symbol on a bright orange sticker identifies a container for possibly infectious material. Red bags or red containers may be substituted for these labels.
- Hold contaminated materials away from your body and handle carefully. Never shake or place these materials in contact with uncontaminated surfaces. Put contaminated materials in a bag or other designated container immediately.

DISPOSAL

- Seal bags of infectious material **when they are only half full.** They will be easier to handle.
- Close bags securely and label according to agency policy.
- Replace the used bag with a clean bag.

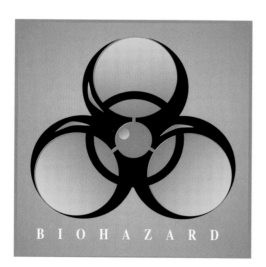

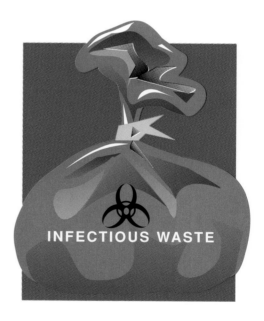

➥ *All used linens are considered contaminated.*
➥ *Once your gloves are contaminated, they will contaminate anything they touch.*

➥ *Your agency may require you to sort contaminated material for reuse (to be cleaned and disinfected) or disposal.*

POINTERS

DOUBLE BAGGING

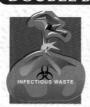

When the outside of a bag of infectious material becomes contaminated, you will place that bag inside a clean bag. One approach is to hold a clean bag open with one hand while one edge of the bag is folded over the back of a chair. With your free hand, pick up the contaminated bag and carefully place it inside the clean one.

DISINFECTANT

To prepare a disinfectant, mix one part household bleach (sodium hypochlorite) with ten parts water. A quick method is:

- Using a fluid measuring cup, put 1/3 cup (2.7 oz.) of bleach in a quart (32 oz.) or liter (33.8 oz.) container. Fill the container with water to nearly full.

- **Use this solution the day you prepare it** as it will lose its power to disinfect.

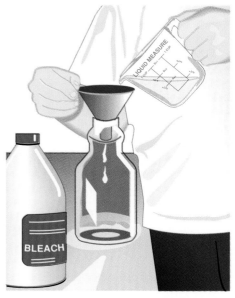

➡ *Bleach-based disinfectant will discolor fabrics and many other materials, including floors. Use carefully, and never leave on surfaces for longer than necessary.*

➡ **Lysol** *is a popular disinfectant available in most grocery stores.*

CLEANING SURFACES

- Clean contaminated surfaces immediately.

- **Always wear gloves.**

- Use clean paper towels (or disposable wipes) and disinfectant.

- Have a plastic bag or container ready for disposal of used towels and gloves.

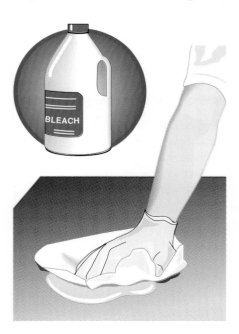

➡ *Never use contaminated materials or equipment again until they have been cleaned according to your agency's policy.*

Completion

*Our **Completion Symbol** reflects our **Preparation Symbol** to emphasize that the practices for completing care are related to the steps and principles of preparation. Use the information on these and the previous pages as a guide whenever you are providing care. When you see the **Completion Symbol**, you will be required to follow these guidelines.*

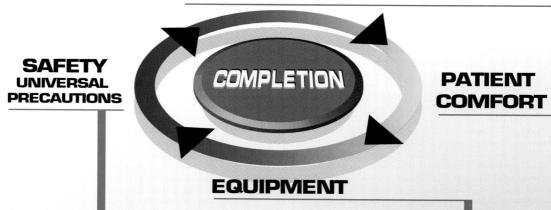

COMMUNICATION

SAFETY
UNIVERSAL PRECAUTIONS

PATIENT COMFORT

EQUIPMENT

Be sensitive to possible hazards to you and the client: contaminated surfaces, conditions that could cause falls, etc.

✔ If using a hospital-type bed, lower bed and position side rails as indicated.

✔ If using removable side rails, replace the side rails as indicated.

✔ Use good body mechanics when lifting or positioning.

✔ Get assistance when you need it: when a client is agitated, if there's an emergency, etc.

✔ **Follow the infection control guidelines on pages 116-123** for handling contaminated materials and equipment.

✔ **Wash your hands.**

Make sure you know what equipment or materials you used and how you should clean, dispose, forward, or store them.

✔ Clean and disinfect all equipment that will be used again, following agency policy. Store in an appropriate area.

✔ Throw away all contaminated disposable materials (including gloves) and equipment, following agency policy.

✔ Follow agency policy on forwarding or laundering soiled linens.

✔ Make a list of any supplies you will need for your next visit.

✔ Follow agency policy for preparing, storing, and forwarding all specimens collected.

✔ Follow agency policy regarding buying and being reimbursed for supplies.

Always maintain the client's right to privacy, dignity, and physical comfort.

✔ Position the client so he or she is comfortable.

✔ Make sure clients are comfortably clothed or covered.

✔ Open curtains.

✔ Adjust lighting and temperature for client comfort.

✔ Ask the client if there is anything else you can do before you leave.

Be clear, accurate, and observant.
Pay attention to the client's feelings.

✔ Tell the client when you are nearing completion of the procedure and when you have finished.

✔ Write information for written records as soon as possible. Never count on your memory.

✔ Be sure to know the difference between what the client tells you (subjective information) and what you observe (objective information).

✔ Tell the client when to expect to see you again.

✔ Immediately report any changes in the client's condition to your supervisor.

Basic Nursing Care

1.
What do you do in a day that you like to do privately? If you were a client, how would you want people to treat your privacy?

2.
What do you do at home to make yourself physically comfortable? Why? Do you think other people have similar habits? Why or why not?

3.
What physical conditions make you uncomfortable? Why? Do you think other people feel the same way? Why or why not?

4.
Make a list of five possible hazards to your safety. How do you think other people should treat your safety? How should you treat theirs? Why?

REVIEW

**Key Terms – Test your understanding of each of these first.
Then use each one once to fill in the incomplete statements below.**

communication

equipment

safety

handwashing

paper towels

gowns or aprons, masks,
and gloves

inside out

biohazard

double bagging

disinfectant

1. Taking Universal Precautions and being alert to potential hazards are necessary for _____ .

2. Gowns, aprons, and masks are turned _____ when removed so that the contaminated side is not showing.

3. Clean contaminated surfaces with _____ .

4. _____ are barriers that are put on in that order when Universal or Isolation Precautions are necessary.

5. _____ is required if the outside of a bag of infectious material becomes contaminated.

6. Vigorous _____ with soap, properly performed, washes off infectious germs and helps prevent their spread.

7. Being clear, accurate, observant, and sensitive to the client are all part of good _____ practice.

8. Use _____ to turn faucets off when handwashing.

9. Always collect the _____ and materials you'll need for a procedure before you begin it.

10. The _____ symbol or a red plastic bag identifies a container for potentially infectious material.

Food & Nutrition

Diets (what people eat) have a direct effect on health.

The goal of diets is to provide the elements of food necessary for health. This is called good **nutrition.** Everyone has basic nutritional needs, but some conditions require special diets. The care plan will indicate the kind of diet your clients are to receive.

You will assist clients to follow a diet by preparing and serving meals.

You may have to prepare meals for a client. This will include purchasing food, preparing it, serving it, and in some cases, feeding it to clients. You will need to understand diets in order to do this.

Eating is both a necessity and an opportunity for pleasure.

You must make sure the client is comfortable, the environment is pleasant, and the food is served the way it was meant to be served (hot, cold, fresh, etc.). Mealtime is an excellent time to talk with clients and ask them about themselves.

Some clients are not able to feed themselves without assistance.

You may have to feed a client, cut his or her food, or just provide special utensils. Because this can be embarrassing or difficult, you will have to be very sensitive to the client's feelings and comfort.

Measuring fluid intake and output is a regular part of maintaining a diet.

Because the body's fluid balance is necessary to health, checking fluid intake and output is an important part of many treatments. When it is, you will be responsible for measuring intake and output.

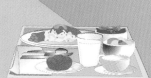

When assisting clients with their nutrition, include these guidelines along with those for preparation and completion on pages 114-115 and 124-125.

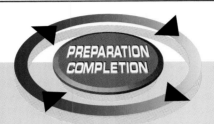

Communication

✔ Make sure you know what foods and how much of them the diet allows, as well as how they are to be prepared.

✔ Ask the client to tell you of any food preferences and try to accommodate them.

✔ Identify the foods on the tray or table for blind or impaired vision clients. Describe the position of the food using clock hour-hand positions: one o'clock, two o'clock, etc.

✔ Take the opportunity to talk with the client during meals.

Client Comfort

✔ Give early notice of meals, allowing time for elimination, hand-washing, and oral hygiene. Assist if appropriate.

✔ Prepare an area that it is neat, clean, and pleasant for eating.

✔ Position the client comfortably in a chair or bed.

✔ Offer to cut the food if clients have difficulty doing it themselves.

✔ Allow clients to take as much time to eat as they like.

✔ If serving a client in bed, place meal trays and between-meal snacks or fluids within easy reach of the client.

✔ Always serve food promptly so that hot food is hot and cold food is cold.

Equipment

✔ Clean and store all pots, pans, dishes, etc. after use.

✔ Be sure to provide any special utensils (such as specially designed forks, knives, spoons, etc.) needed by the client.

Safety

✔ When cooking, never leave the stove unattended.

✔ Make sure food and fluids are never hot enough to burn.

✔ Refrigerate and store foods properly to prevent spoiling.

Basic Nutrition

> **Nutrients are the elements of food which the body uses for energy, maintenance, healing, and growth.**

Proteins, carbohydrates, fats, vitamins, and minerals are the five types of nutrients needed by the body. The body's use of these from food is called nutrition.

> **The basic elements of good nutrition are nutrients, fluids, and fiber.**

Everyone needs balanced amounts of these elements for their body to function properly. Too little of any of these elements will have a negative effect on health. Too much can also cause problems.

> **The average adult needs approximately 2.5 liters of water daily.**

Water is the most important element in the body and makes up about two-thirds of each person's body weight. It helps control the body's temperature by distributing heat evenly throughout the body and releasing it through perspiration. It is also necessary for the body's process of eliminating waste. If the body loses too much water **(dehydration)** or doesn't lose enough **(edema)**, it can have serious results, including death.

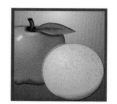 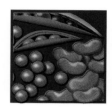

The

PROTEINS

Main sources: meat, fish, eggs, dairy products, peas, beans.
Necessary for the growth of muscle and other body tissue.

CARBOHYDRATES

Main sources: grains, cereal, bread, potatoes, peas, beans.
Complex carbohydrates are the best and primary source of energy for the body.

FIBER

Main sources: cereals, grains, fruit, vegetables.
Aids the body in digestion and in eliminating waste.

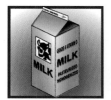 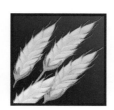 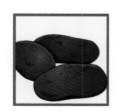 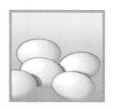 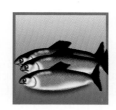 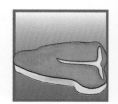

Elements Of Good Nutrition

FATS

Main sources: meat, dairy products, vegetable oils, egg yolks.
While too much fat is bad for health, some fat is necessary. Fat in the body helps maintain body warmth, stores certain vitamins, and is a source of energy.

VITAMINS

Main sources: fruit, vegetables, meat, dairy products.
Complex chemicals important to the functioning of various body systems (the liver, muscles, bone growth, etc.).

WATER

Main sources: food and liquids.
Almost half of the body's need for water comes from food intake and the other half from fluid intake. Fluid intake and output should be equal, though only about 40% of fluid output is urine. Most of the rest is lost in evaporation.

MINERALS

Main sources: fruit, vegetables, meat, fish, dairy products, grains.
Substances such as calcium for bone growth and strength, iron for blood, iodine for the thyroid, etc.

The Balanced Diet

Balancing food groups is a useful way to have balanced nutrition.

To have a balanced diet, the United States Department of Agriculture (USDA) traditionally recommended including in the diet food from four basic groups: milk and dairy products, meat and fish, vegetables and fruit, and bread and cereals. It now recommends balancing foods from *five basic groups* described at right, while *using a sixth group (fats, oils, and sweets) sparingly.*

The type and amount of food are important elements in a diet.

Calories are the amount of energy in food that will be released when it is used by the body. Everyone needs a certain amount of calories in their diet, though this amount will differ by size, weight, age, and other factors. The Food Guide Pyramid at right recommends numbers of servings that will both balance the diet and provide the necessary calories.

The type and amount of nutrients, fluids, and fiber can differ widely within a food group.

A one-time substitution of one food in a group for another may or may not result in the same amount of nutrition. Over a period of time, however, a balance of different foods from within each group should result in balanced nutrition.

There is no universal diet.

The pyramid recommended by the USDA shows a general way to have a balanced diet. Learning it should help you better understand, prepare, and explain the diets you serve to clients.

SERVING SIZES

The number of recommended daily servings will be different for each person. Those shown in the pyramid are *average* recommendations. Here are some sample serving sizes recommended by the USDA:

Food	# of Servings
1 slice of bread	1
1 tortilla	1
1/2 cup cooked rice or pasta	1
1 oz. of cereal	1
1/2 cup cooked vegetables	1
1 cup leafy vegetables	1
1/2 cup scalloped potatoes	1
10 french fries	1
Apple, orange, or banana	1
1/2 cup canned fruit	1
3/4 cup fruit juice	1
1 cup milk (skim, low-fat, whole)	1
8 oz. of yogurt	1
1.5 oz. cheddar cheese	1
2 oz. processed cheese	1
1/2 cup ice cream	1
2-3 oz. lean meat, poultry, fish	1
3 oz. hamburger	1
1 egg	1
1/2 cup dry beans or peas	1
2 tablespoons of peanut butter	1

THE FOOD GUIDE PYRAMID

At the bottom of the Pyramid, are the foods you need the most in your diet. As you go up the Pyramid, you need less.

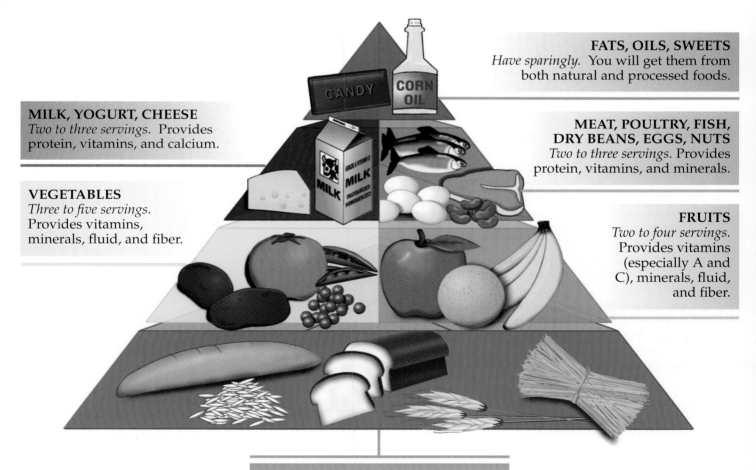

FATS, OILS, SWEETS
Have sparingly. You will get them from both natural and processed foods.

MILK, YOGURT, CHEESE
Two to three servings. Provides protein, vitamins, and calcium.

MEAT, POULTRY, FISH, DRY BEANS, EGGS, NUTS
Two to three servings. Provides protein, vitamins, and minerals.

VEGETABLES
Three to five servings. Provides vitamins, minerals, fluid, and fiber.

FRUITS
Two to four servings. Provides vitamins (especially A and C), minerals, fluid, and fiber.

BREADS, CEREALS, RICE, PASTA
Six to eleven servings. Provides complex carbohydrates, vitamins, minerals, and fiber.

Client Diets

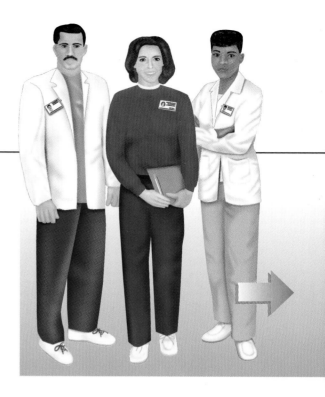

Diets are an important part of care.

You will be given specific instructions regarding the kind of diet to be served to clients. The *general* diet served to most clients is a balanced diet.

Many clients require special diets as part of their treatment.

Clients with heart problems, allergies, diabetes, fever, and who have had surgery are among those that require special diets. Since mistakes on special diets can have serious results, you must always make sure the client is getting the correct diet. If you are unsure about anything regarding a special diet, discuss it with your supervisor.

Measuring dietary intake and output (I&O) is an important way to check a client's condition.

Each person's intake and output should balance. For this and other reasons, you will often be required to check food and fluid intake and output (feces, urine, vomitus). This will include measuring fluid intake and urine output. Your report of these observations and measurements *must be accurate.* It will be used by the home care team to assess the client's condition and treatment.

RESPONSIBILITIES OF THE HOME CARE AIDE

✔ Preparing and serving the client's diet, including special diets.

✔ Ensuring that the client is getting the correct diet.

✔ Reporting the client's dietary intake and output.

CLEAR LIQUID:

Water, tea, apple juice, black coffee, clear broth, and other clear fluids.

For clients with acute nausea and vomiting.

FULL LIQUID:

All liquids, including strained soups, milk, ice cream, and other non-clear liquids.

For clients graduating from clear liquid diet, or with sensitive digestion, or difficulty chewing.

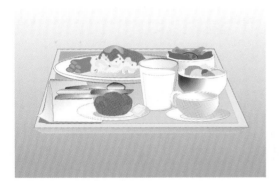

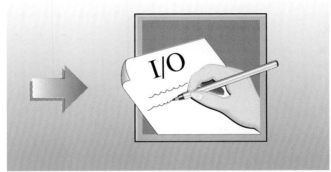

THE CLIENT'S DIET
• GENERAL DIET •

A balance of nutrients, fluids, and fiber.
For most clients.

REPORTING INTAKE AND OUTPUT

SOME SPECIAL DIETS

SOFT:

All liquids, cooked vegetables, ground meat, fish, pureed solids, and other soft foods.

For clients graduating from full liquid diet, sensitive digestion, infections, and certain other disorders.

RESTRICTED SODIUM (Salt):

Less salt is used in preparing food and no salt is allowed to be added by the client. Condiments and other additives containing salt (ketchup, mustard, margarine, etc.) may also be prohibited.

For clients with heart disease and certain other disorders.

LOW-FAT:

Lean meats, poultry, pasta, breads, cereals, vegetables and other low-fat or fat-free foods.

For clients with heart disease, high cholesterol and certain other disorders.

DIABETIC:

Carbohydrates, fats, and proteins are carefully prescribed by the physician.

For clients with diabetes mellitus.

HIGH-PROTEIN:

Meat, fish, eggs, dairy products, and other high protein foods.

For clients needing protein for tissue growth.

Meal Preparation

Preparing meals is one of the most common tasks noted in care plans. Home care aides are regularly required to provide clients with nutritious, pleasant, and satisfying meals. Your agency and supervisor will inform you of your meal preparation responsibilities and guidelines for each client. You will not be expected to master the many different styles of cooking that reflect cultural and individual preferences, but will be required to meet the client's basic nutritional needs.

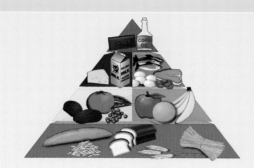

1. PLAN A MENU

menu: a list of the foods and liquids served at a meal.
appetizing: stimulating to the appetite; delicious.

The first step in meal preparation is to plan a *menu*. Your menu should reflect the following:

- a balanced diet (or special diets, if ordered);
- client preferences, whenever possible;
- affordability;
- your ability to prepare it within a reasonable time;
- a regular meal schedule;
- an appetizing meal;
- your supervisor's instructions and agency guidelines.

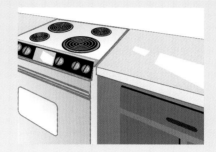

2. PREPARE THE KITCHEN

Preparing a meal requires handling different activities at the same time. This will be easier if:

- the kitchen is neat and clean;
- all dishes and cookware are clean and ready for use;
- you have a clean and open surface on which to work;
- all necessary appliances (toasters, blenders, food processors, etc.) are accessible and ready for use.

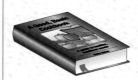

It's worthwhile to buy yourself a good basic cookbook both for work and personal use. It will provide you with recipes, menu tips, practical procedures, and information on ingredients and serving sizes.

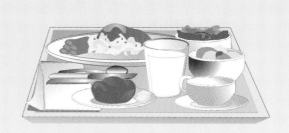

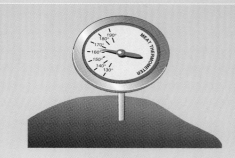

3. PREPARE FOOD

- Wash your hands before you handle food. If you interrupt food preparation for another activity, wash your hands before handling food again.
- Collect the ingredients you will need. Make sure the ingredients reflect the client's dietary requirements or restrictions.
- Prepare ingredients that will spoil at room temperature last. Foods that require refrigeration should not be left at room temperature for any longer than necessary.
- Use the proper cookware and appliances. For example: only use microwave safe cookware in a microwave; don't use a toaster oven for a roast; etc.
- Never leave the stove unattended during cooking or an appliance that is on (blender, microwave, etc.). This is both for safety and for meal quality.
- Use pot holders to handle cookware.

FOOD SAFETY

It is important to handle, prepare, and store foods properly to avoid spoiling and possible food poisoning.

- Never undercook meat. A food temperature of 165° is necessary to kill bacteria found in meat. You can use a meat thermometer to test this.
- Foods that will spoil should be prepared as quickly as possible.
- Frozen foods that can spoil at room temperature should be thawed as quickly as possible and cooked *before* they come to room temperature.
- Keep uncooked fresh foods *separate* (meat from fish from eggs, etc.) to avoid spreading bacteria from one food to another. Use different surfaces and utensils to prepare different types of uncooked fresh foods.
- Refrigeration should be below 45° to prevent spoiling.
- Cover unserved portions to prevent bacterial contamination.
- When storing leftovers, cool quickly by only partially covering. Refrigerate in small containers.

Serving a Meal

When serving a meal, you must prepare an area that is neat, clean, and pleasant for eating. Allow time for the client to prepare and perform personal care before the meal. Never rush the client and always be friendly, helpful, and accommodating. Your manner and actions will help determine the client's meal experience.

1. PREPARATION

- Follow the preparation guidelines on pages 114-115 as indicated by the Preparation Symbol. Pay special attention to the guidelines on *Food & Nutrition* on page 129.
- Wash your hands.
- Prepare an area for the meal that is neat, clean, and pleasant. Make sure the client is comfortably positioned in a chair or in bed.

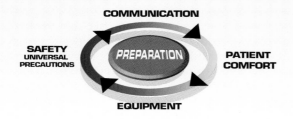

EQUIPMENT

- special utensils if appropriate (see pages 274-275 on *Assistive Devices*).

2. ASSEMBLE THE MEAL

- Collect dishes, utensils, glasses, and napkins. Provide salt, pepper, and condiments **if the diet allows them.**
- Serve portions of food and liquids appropriate to the client. Make sure you serve **all** the food and liquids you are supposed to serve.

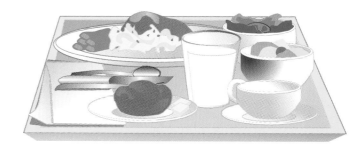

➡ *Special utensils help clients with physical disabilities to eat without assistance. They often have specially designed handles for holding the utensil. There are also specially designed cups, glasses, and dishes.*

➡ *Serve food promptly so that hot food is hot and cold food is cold.*

➡ **When serving a special diet, never add salt, sugar, or condiments without checking with your supervisor.**

POINTERS

138

MEAL PRESENTATION

✔ Meals should be attractively presented. Foods should have different color and texture. They should never be thrown together on a plate. Provide separate dishes for foods which clients want separate (salads, for example).

✔ Provide a pleasant atmosphere for the meal. Never work around the client while he or she is eating.

3. IDENTIFY FOOD

● Position the meal in easy reach of the client. Describe food in positive terms that indicate you think it is appetizing.

● Identify the foods on the tray for blind or impaired vision clients using clock hour-hand positions: one o'clock, two o'clock, etc.

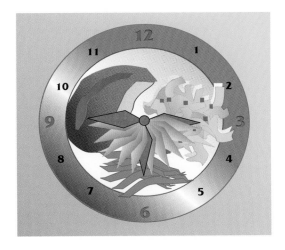

4. PREPARE FOOD

● For clients with physical disabilities, offer to cut food, butter bread, and open cartons and other packaging.

● If you have other tasks to perform, you may do them now but return in 10-15 minutes to check on the client. When he or she is finished, measure and record intake if indicated and remove the dishes.

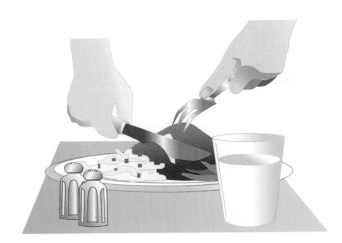

➦ *Your attitude about the client's diet will make an impression on the client. Be positive.*

Follow the completion guidelines on pages 124-125 as indicated by the Completion Symbol. Pay special attention to the guidelines on *Food & Nutrition* on page 129.

Feeding a Client

You may have to feed some clients who are unable to feed themselves. Such clients may feel helpless and become frustrated, embarrassed, angry, etc. as a result. They are especially dependent upon you to make eating a pleasurable experience. Talk with them and allow them to take as much time to eat as they like. Allow them as much control as possible over their mealtime. Always be considerate, attentive, and sensitive.

PROCEDURE

1. PREPARATION

- Follow the preparation guidelines on pages 114-115 as indicated by the Preparation Symbol. Pay special attention to the guidelines on *Food & Nutrition* on page 129.

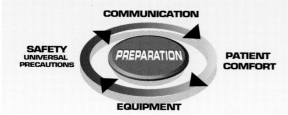

- Wash your hands. Prepare an area for the meal. Make sure the client is comfortably positioned. If in bed, the client must be raised to a sitting position.

- Assemble the meal. Make sure you serve everything that is supposed to be served.

2. PREPARE FOOD

- Place a napkin under the client's chin across the chest.

- Position the meal before the client and identify the food in it.

- Cut food, butter bread, and open cartons. If allowed, add seasoning or condiments requested by the client.

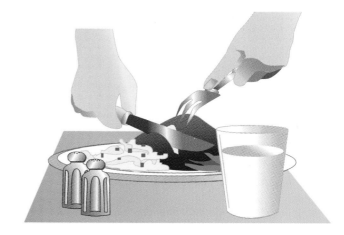

➡ *With some clients or meals, you may want to place a towel over the client's chest as additional protection before you place the napkin.*

➡ *Food should be cut into small teaspoon-size pieces.*

➡ *It is generally a good idea for the client to try a food before adding seasoning.*

POINTERS

3. SERVE

- Serve each food one bite at a time using a spoon two-thirds full. Ask the client to indicate which food or fluid he or she wants next.

- Offer liquids routinely. If the client prefers to use a straw, use different straws for each liquid.

- **Allow hot liquids to cool.** Stir them to cool faster.

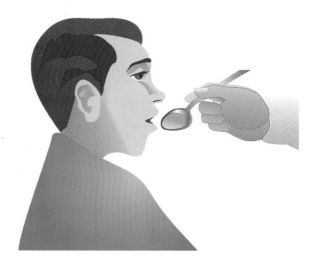

➡ *Never rush the client. Allow time for chewing and swallowing.*

➡ *Too much of one thing (especially liquids) can cause the client to feel full. If you balance each food as you go, the client will get a balanced meal even if he or she does not finish.*

4. COMPLETE

- Wipe around the client's mouth with a napkin as needed.

- When finished, remove the tray and position client comfortably. Measure intake if indicated. Report any difficulties with swallowing *(dysphagia)*, appetite, etc.

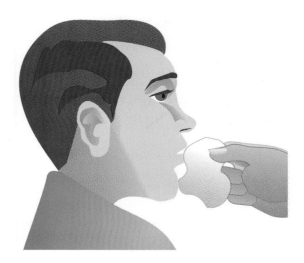

Follow the completion guidelines on pages 124-125 as indicated by the Completion Symbol. Pay special attention to the guidelines on *Food & Nutrition* on page 129.

Fluid Intake and Output (I&O)

Measuring fluid intake and output is a regular part of checking a client's condition.

To maintain homeostasis, the body must take in and put out an equal amount of water each day. Failure to keep a proper fluid balance is a sign of a serious disorder that must be watched and treated.

To determine fluid intake, you will measure the amount of fluid clients take in from the food and fluids you serve them.

The sources of water in the diet that are easiest to measure are fluids (water, milk, juice, soups, etc.) and soft foods such as ice cream, pudding, and jello. The amounts of all fluids served are recorded as they are served. Leftover fluids are then subtracted from the amounts served. The resulting amount is recorded on the I&O record as intake. To make this easier, you may want to *pre-measure containers* for serving fluids using a measuring cup.

To determine output, you will measure the amount of fluid clients put out in urine and other body fluids.

Urine represents about 40% of average fluid output and is generally what you will measure. Vomitus and wound drainage are sometimes measured, while diarrhea is generally just noted and reported.

You will use a liquid measuring cup to measure I&O.

The measuring cup should be marked in ounces (oz) and milliliters (ml) or cubic centimeters (cc). There are 30 milliliters or cubic centimeters in one ounce. You will measure intake and output in *different measuring cups* and you will record the result in milliliters or cubic centimeters on the I&O record.

MEASURING INTAKE

- Measure serving amounts. See above note on *Pre-Measuring Serving Containers.*
- When the client finishes the meal, pour leftover liquids into **the measuring cup reserved for intake.** Measure one liquid at a time.
- Measure amounts at your eye level. Hold the measuring cup level so there is no distortion.
- Subtract leftover amounts from amounts served. Follow your agency's policy for recording the amounts on the I&O record.

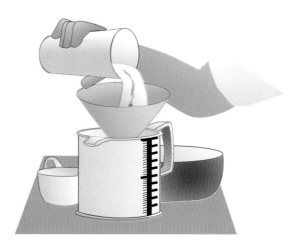

➡ *Dry measure cups are not the same as liquid measuring cups. Dry measures come in fraction of a cup sizes (1/3, 1/4, etc.). You must use a liquid measuring cup.*

➡ *When fluids are spilled, you will have to estimate how much has been spilled and subtract that from the serving amount.*

PRE-MEASURING SERVING CONTAINERS

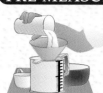

Pre-measuring serving containers for drinks, soups, and other liquids can save time and simplify your measurements. To do so, pour water into the container to a normal serving level. Then pour the water into the measuring cup. Make a list of the measurements and keep it handy in the kitchen.

MEASURING OUTPUT

- **Observe Universal Precautions. Put on disposable gloves.** Pour urine from the bedpan, urinal, drainage bag, etc. into **the measuring cup reserved for output.**

- Measure amounts at your eye level. Hold the measuring cup level so there is no distortion.

- Dispose of urine and clean all equipment. Remove gloves and wash hands. Follow your agency's policy for recording the amount on the I&O record.

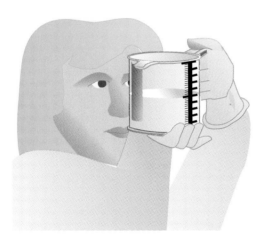

➡ *Clients whose I&O is measured urinate into a bedpan, commode, or urinal (not a toilet). Used toilet tissue is thrown away separately and not put in with the urine.*

➡ *You may have to estimate urine lost through incontinence. The client can help you, though you must be sensitive to his or her possible embarrassment.*

I&O RECORD

- Follow your agency's policy for reporting (see pages 28-29). Use a pen and write clearly.

- **Record amounts at the time they are consumed or eliminated. Don't wait.**

- Measurements are in cubic centimeters (cc) or milliliters (ml), according to your agency's policy. (1 oz=30cc. 1cc=1ml.)

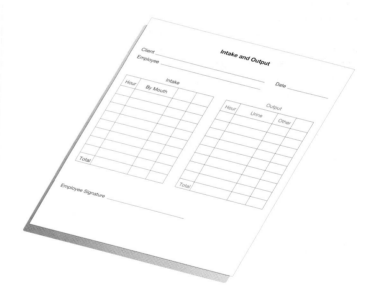

➡ *The intake and output sheet should be kept in a handy and visible location.*

Food & Nutrition

1.
Consider the importance meals have for you in addition to providing nutrition: sensory pleasure, socializing, celebrating, etc. What are the aspects of meals that you enjoy most. Why?

2.
Consider what it would be like to be put on the special diets described on pages 134-135. How would you feel about it? Why?

3.
If you *had* to be fed by someone, how would it affect how you enjoyed a meal?

4.
When you are being served food, what likes and dislikes do you have?

REVIEW

**Key Terms – Test your understanding of each of these first.
Then use each one once to fill in the incomplete statements below.**

diets

water

fluid balance

hot food

fluid intake

fluid output

liquid measuring cup

room temperature

165°

45°

1. To maintain homeostasis, the body must maintain proper _____.

2. Foods that require refrigeration should not be left at _____ _____ any longer than is necessary.

3. Meats should be cooked to a temperature of _____ to kill bacteria.

4. You will measure output with a _____, marked in ounces (oz) and milliliters (ml) or cubic centimeters (cc).

5. The most measurable sources of _____ are fluids (water, milk, juice, soups, etc.) and soft foods such as ice cream, pudding, and jello.

6. You must always serve food promptly so that _____ is hot and cold food is cold.

7. _____ (what people eat) have a direct effect on health.

8. Refrigeration should be below _____ to keep food from spoiling.

9. Urine represents about 40% of average _____ and is the form that is generally measured.

10. The most important element in the body is _____.

Bedmaking

The condition of the client's bed is an important element in his or her experience of home care.

Clients who need bedrest spend most of their time in bed, and all clients spend a large amount of time in bed, even if only to sleep.

A neat, clean, and well-made bed provides comfort and prevents a number of problems.

The condition of the bed can have physical and psychological effects upon a client. A poorly made bed can irritate a client's skin and lead to bedsores. A bed contaminated by body fluids can help spread contagious disease. Sloppy or soiled bed linens can also embarrass clients, especially when they have visitors.

You will make both unoccupied and occupied beds.

It is much easier to make a bed without a client in it (unoccupied). However, making a bed with the client still in it (occupied) is often necessary for health and safety reasons. When doing so, be especially sensitive to the client's concerns.

You will have to handle soiled and potentially infectious bed linens.

Universal Precautions are required if there are any blood, semen, vaginal secretions, or any body fluids (feces, urine, vomitus, etc.) in which you can see blood. Follow your agency's policy on bedmaking and the guidelines presented in this unit to protect the safety and comfort of your clients and yourself.

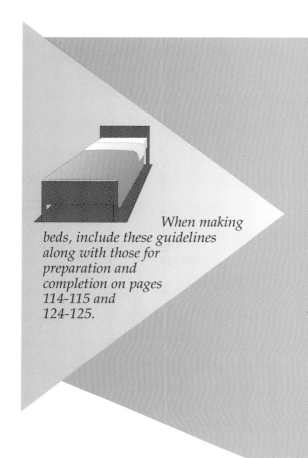

When making beds, include these guidelines along with those for preparation and completion on pages 114-115 and 124-125.

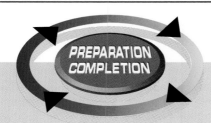

PREPARATION COMPLETION

Communication
✔ When making an occupied bed, speak clearly. The client needs to be able to follow your directions.

Client Comfort
✔ Change linens regularly (at least once a week) so they remain clean and fresh.

✔ When making an occupied bed, be especially sensitive to privacy, personal dignity, and physical comfort.

✔ The bed linens on which the client lies must be tight and smooth, without any wrinkles or lumps.

Equipment
✔ Collect the linen you will need.

✔ Any linens not being changed (mattress pad, plastic draw sheet, blanket, bed spread, top sheet) should be folded for easy reuse and placed on a clean surface.

Safety
✔ Hold clean bed linens away from your body so they are not contaminated by your uniform. Be sure to place them on a clean surface while you make the bed.

✔ If using a hospital-type bed, raise the bed to a comfortable height for you to work. This lessens back strain.(See note below on *Hospital Beds*.)

✔ Make sure the client is always protected from falling out of bed any time you are making an occupied bed.

✔ Wearing gloves, change the linens immediately any time the bed has been contaminated by body fluids (often from an incontinent client).

✔ Always roll dirty linen away from you. Hold it away from your uniform and never shake it.

✔ Practice *Universal Precautions* any time you might come in contact with any blood or body fluids (feces, urine, vomitus, etc.).

HOSPITAL BEDS

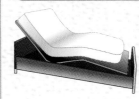

Many clients who spend a lot of time in bed use an adjustable hospital-type bed. These beds allow you to adjust the height and position of the bed and may have attached side rails. Read the manufacturer's directions on how to operate the bed.

Making an Unoccupied Bed

The unoccupied bed is made one side at a time for efficiency and ease. The linens are tucked in tightly and smoothly using *mitered corners*. When finished, the bed is left either *open* or *closed*.

PROCEDURE

1. PREPARATION

- Follow the preparation guidelines on pages 114-115 as indicated by the Preparation Symbol. Pay special attention to the guidelines on *Bedmaking* on page 147.

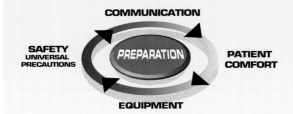

- Ask your clients about any preferences they have about how to make their beds.

EQUIPMENT

Bed Linens
- mattress pad
- bottom sheet
- plastic draw sheet (if indicated)
- cotton draw sheet (if indicated)
- top sheet
- blanket
- bedspread
- pillowcases

➡ *Collect the linens you need in the order you will use them, with the mattress pad first. Then turn them over so the mattress pad is on top.*

➡ *Place the linens on a clean surface (the back of a chair, for example) while you are making the bed.*

2. APPLY BOTTOM LINENS

- Unfold the mattress pad so that it is even with the top edge of the mattress.
- Unfold the bottom sheet so that it is even with the bottom edge of the mattress and hangs over the head and side of the bed. Its center fold should be at the center of the mattress.
- Fan-fold the top fold of the sheet to the other side of the bed.

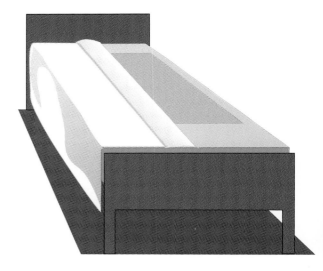

➡ *Fan folding means to fold back in small folds that sit on each other, looking like the folds of a fan.*

➡ *The large hem of the sheet is at the head of the bed and the hem stitching is placed face down so it won't irritate the client's skin.*

POINTERS

REMOVING LINENS

Before making an unoccupied bed, you will usually have to remove soiled bed linens. **Always roll soiled linens away from you. Hold them away from your uniform and never shake them.** Put soiled linens where directed by your supervisor and the client. The mattress pad, plastic draw sheet, blanket, and bed spread may be reused if they are not soiled or contaminated by body fluids. Any linens being reused should be handled according to the guidelines on page 153.

3. MAKE MITERED CORNERS

- Tightly tuck the top of the sheet under the head of the mattress.
- Grasp the edge of the sheet about 10 inches from the corner and fold it over the mattress, forming a triangle (# 1 & 2).
- Tuck the hanging corner of the sheet under the mattress (#3).
- Lower the side of the sheet and tuck it tightly under the side of the mattress (#4).

4. POSITION DRAW SHEET

- Unfold the plastic draw sheet so that it is about fifteen inches from the top edge of the mattress and its center fold is at the center of the mattress. Fan-fold the top fold of the sheet to the other side of the bed.
- Repeat the procedure with the cotton draw sheet, placing it directly over the plastic sheet. Tuck both tightly under the side of the mattress.

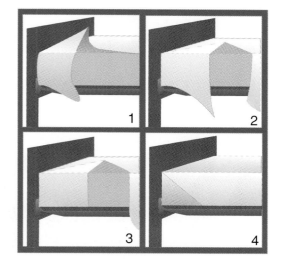

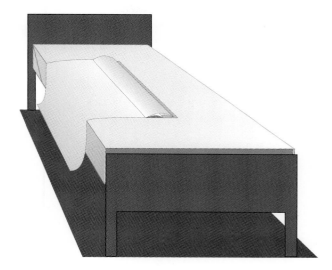

➡ *Be careful not to let the sheet touch the floor as you unfold it.*

➡ *Smooth the linens as you go.*

➡ *Plastic draw sheets must be completely covered by a cotton draw sheet.*

Making an Unoccupied Bed (Cont'd)

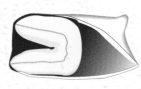

PILLOWS

Put pillows in their cases by folding the pillow in half lengthwise and slipping it into the case. Place the pillow on the bed with the open end *away* from the door to the room. Always be careful not to contaminate the pillow or case by allowing contact with any unclean surfaces.

PROCEDURE

5. FINISH BOTTOM LINENS

- Move to the other side of the bed and repeat steps 3, 4, and 5. Begin by unfolding the fan-folded bottom sheet and tucking it in using a mitered corner at the head of the bed.

- Tuck in the plastic and cotton draw sheets.

6. POSITION TOP SHEET

- Unfold the top sheet so that the large hem is even with the top edge of the mattress and the bottom of the sheet hangs over the foot of the bed. The hem stitching should face up.

- Fan-fold the sheet to the other side of the bed.

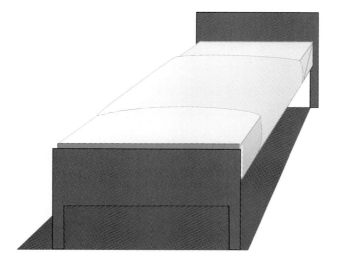

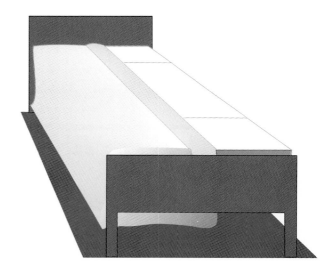

➥ *Make sure the linens are tucked in tightly and wrinkle free.*

➥ *There are different practices for using draw sheets. Follow your agency's practice.*

POINTERS

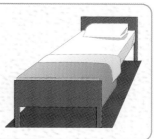

THE OPEN BED

Step 8, below, is for making a closed bed. If you are asked to make an *open bed*, fan-fold back the top linens (top sheet, blanket, and bedspread) to about 24 inches from the foot of the bed. The top fold is covered by the top sheet with its wide hem showing.

7. APPLY BLANKET AND BEDSPREAD

- Repeat the procedure with a blanket and, if used, a bedspread. The top of the blanket is placed about six inches from the top edge of the mattress, while a bedspread is placed so it meets the mattress's top edge.

- Tuck the top sheet, blanket, and bedspread together under the foot of the mattress. **Make a mitered corner, but do not tuck in the sides.**

8. COMPLETION

- Move to the other side of the bed and repeat steps 6 & 7.

- Fold the top edge of the bedspread under the blanket and then fold the sheet over it to make a neat cuff.

- Put the pillow in the pillowcase (see note on p. 150). Place on the bed with the open end away from the door.

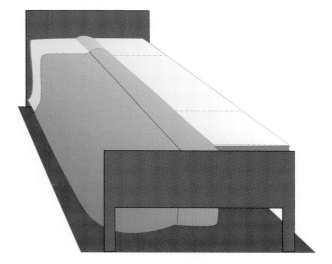

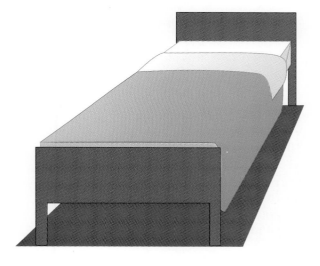

➡ *There are many different approaches to positioning a bedspread. Ask your client how he or she would like it.*

Follow the completion guidelines on pages 124-125 as indicated by the Completion Symbol. Pay special attention to the guidelines on *Bedmaking* on page 147.

Making an Occupied Bed

Home care aides make an occupied bed when clients are confined to bed. The client is covered with a bath blanket and turned to the far side while you remove the soiled bottom linens and make that side of the bed. You then roll the client over the fan-folded bottom linens onto his or her other side and complete making the other side of the bed. Clients confined to bed will often use *side rails.* See the note regarding side rails on page 154.

PROCEDURE

1. PREPARATION

- Follow the preparation guidelines on pages 114-115 as indicated by the Preparation Symbol. Pay special attention to the guidelines on *Bedmaking* on page 147 and on *Turning a Client* on pages 166-167.

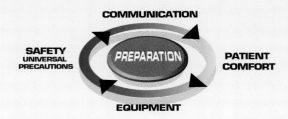

- Ask your clients about any preferences they have about how to make their beds.

EQUIPMENT

Bed Linens
- bottom sheet
- plastic draw sheet (if indicated)
- cotton draw sheet (if indicated)
- top sheet
- blanket
- bedspread
- pillowcases
- bath blanket

➡ *Collect the linens you need in the order you will use them. Then turn them over so the bottom sheet is on top.*

➡ *Place the linens on a clean surface while you are making the bed.*

2. REMOVE TOP LINENS

- Pull out the tucked-in top-sheet, blanket, and bedspread from under the foot of the mattress. Remove the bedspread and blanket, folding them back neatly if you are going to re-use them.

- Cover the top sheet with the bath blanket. Ask the client to grasp the bath blanket while you remove the top sheet.

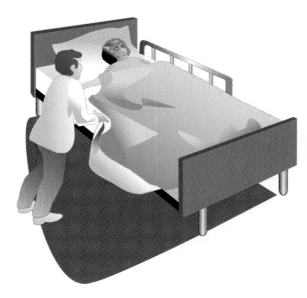

➡ *Make sure the mattress is positioned at the head of the bed.*

➡ *If using side rails, lower or remove the rail on the side you will work first and make sure the opposite rail is raised.*

POINTERS

REUSING BED LINENS

When being reused, the mattress pad remains on the bed and is smoothed out. The plastic draw sheet, blanket, and bedspread are removed by folding each item in half from top to bottom, then from side to side, and then from top to bottom again. Place each on a clean surface (the back of a chair, for example) while you work.

---

3. REMOVE BOTTOM LINENS

- Turn the client to the far side of the bed. He or she may grasp the side rail for support if one is used.
- Pull out the tucked-in draw sheets and bottom sheet from the head to the foot of the mattress.
- Fan-fold the bottom linens snugly against the client's back. Smooth out the exposed mattress pad.

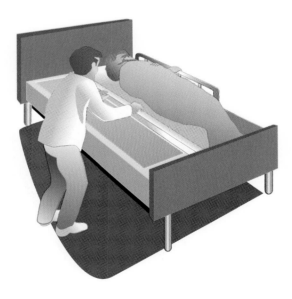

➡ *Be alert to incontinence and put on disposable gloves immediately if the client has soiled the linens with body fluids.*

➡ *Reposition the pillow for comfort and support.*

4. REPLACE BOTTOM SHEET

- Unfold the clean bottom sheet over the mattress pad so that the center fold of the sheet is at the center of the mattress. The sheet should be even with the bottom edge of the mattress and hang over the head and side of the bed.
- Fan-fold the top fold of the sheet to the client's back.
- Tuck the top and side of the sheet under the mattress using a mitered corner (see step 3 on page 149).

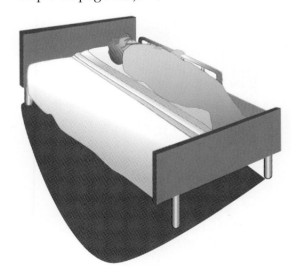

➡ *The large hem of the sheet is at the head of the bed and the hem stitching is placed face down so it won't irritate the client's skin.*

Making an Occupied Bed (Cont'd)

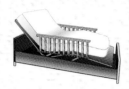
PROCEDURE

5. REPLACE DRAW SHEETS

- If a plastic draw sheet is used, unfold it so it is about fifteen inches below the top edge of the mattress and the center fold is at the center of the mattress. Fan-fold the top fold of the sheet to the client's back.

- Repeat the procedure with the cotton draw sheet, placing it directly over the plastic sheet. Tuck both tightly under the side of the mattress and raise or replace the side rail.

6. REPEAT ON OTHER SIDE

- Move to the other side of the bed and repeat steps 3, 4, and 5. Begin by lowering or removing the side rail and rolling the client over the fan-folded linens to the far side of the bed.

- Remove the soiled bottom linens and place in the linen hamper. Roll soiled linens away from you from the head to the foot of the bed.

- Unfold and tuck in the bottom sheet and then the draw sheets.

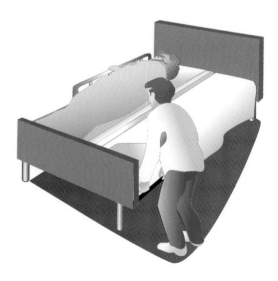

➡ *Smooth the linens as you go.*

➡ *If the plastic draw sheet is being re-used, you will unfold the fan-folded sheet back over the clean bottom sheet.*

➡ *Pull the bottom linens firmly toward you before tucking in to make sure they are tight and wrinkle free.*

POINTERS

7. APPLY TOP SHEET

- Place the client in his or her back in the center of the bed. Raise or replace the side rail if one is used.
- Unfold the clean top sheet over the bath blanket so that the sheet is centered on the bed and the large hem is even with the top edge of the mattress. The hem stitching should face up.
- Ask the client to grasp the top sheet while you remove the bath blanket.

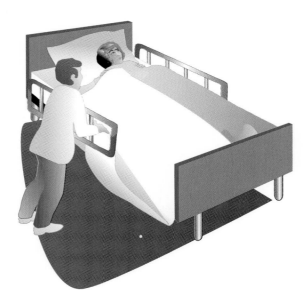

➡ *Roll the bath blanket away from you from the head to the foot of the bed.*

8. COMPLETION

- Unfold the blanket so it is about six inches from the top edge of the mattress. Unfold the bedspread so it reaches the top of the mattress. Fold the top edge of the bedspread under the blanket and then fold the sheet over it to make a neat cuff.
- Smooth the top linens and tuck together under the foot of the mattress, using mitered corners on each side.
- Change the pillowcase (see p.150).

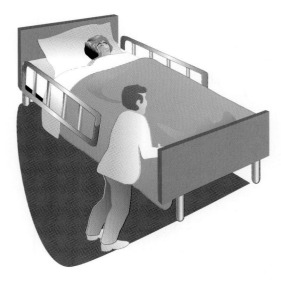

Follow the completion guidelines on pages 124-125 as indicated by the Completion Symbol. Pay special attention to the guidelines on *Bedmaking* on page 147.

Bedmaking

1.
What are your likes and dislikes about the way your bed is made?

2.
Imagine that you are confined to bed. What concerns (privacy, comfort, etc.) would you have about having your bed made while you are in it?

3.
List all the safety issues you can think of in making unoccupied and occupied beds. Consider client safety and your own.

4.
What do you think are the most important things to remember about bedmaking?

REVIEW

**Key Terms – Test your understanding of each of these first.
Then use each one once to fill in the incomplete statements below.**

bed condition

unoccupied bed

occupied bed

clean linens

mitered corner

incontinence

soiled linen

mattress pad

closed bed

open bed

1. Always roll _____ away from you and dispose immediately into a linen hamper or other appropriate container.

2. A _____ is always used to tuck in bed linens.

3. The _____ is left on the bed and smoothed out when being reused.

4. When making an _____ , you have to be especially sensitive to protecting the client's privacy and personal dignity.

5. The top linens cover the bed in a _____. They are fan-folded to the foot of the bed in an _____.

6. _____ should be gathered in the order you will use them and carefully placed on a clean surface while you are making the bed.

7. The _____ can have a physical and psychological impact on the client.

8. _____ causes body fluid contamination of bed linens, requiring you to use universal precautions and to change the linens immediately.

9. An _____ is easier to make than an occupied one.

Positioning a Client in Bed

Positioning clients in bed is a regular responsibility of the home care aide. You will have to reposition clients undergoing bedrest often to prevent the development of pressure sores (decubitus ulcers), contractures, and other problems. Many procedures also require specific positioning of clients confined to bed.

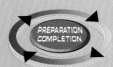

When positioning the client in bed, include these guidelines along with those for preparation and completion on pages 114-115 and 124-125.

Client Comfort

✔ Use pillows to support and cushion the client. Make sure he or she is comfortable.

✔ Be sensitive. The client may be embarrassed to need your assistance.

Communication

✔ Speak clearly. Clients need to be able to follow your directions.

✔ Ask clients to tell you anytime they don't feel well or are uncomfortable.

✔ Tell the client you will help him or her to move on a count of three.

Equipment

✔ If using a hospital-type bed, follow manufacturer's instructions for use. Position the bed at a height that will be comfortable for you to work. It should be as close to waist high as possible so you won't have to bend. Lower it to the proper position when done.

✔ Make adjustments for IV's or catheters.

Safety

✔ **Check for any position restrictions.** Some clients will not be allowed to be placed in some positions.

✔ Lock bed wheels if there are any. Use side rails as indicated.

✔ Always use good body mechanics (see pages 92-93). Bend your legs, not your back. Don't lean or reach.

✔ Never attempt to reposition a client by yourself unless you are certain you can do so easily. Report any positioning difficulty to your supervisor.

✔ Know which clients can help and which can't.

✔ Be careful to avoid friction to the client's skin from sliding on sheets. When repositioning, check the client's skin condition for pale or reddened areas.

See the notes on page 147 regarding hospital-type beds and on 154 regarding side rails.

FOWLER'S POSITION

- The client is positioned between 45 and 60 degrees by using pillows or raising the head of adjustable beds. A *Semi-Fowler* position is raised about 30 degrees. Because the upper body is raised, it is important to keep the client's spine straight. Pillows are placed under the head and knees or arms.

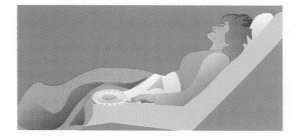

SUPINE

- The client lies flat on his or her back. The head is supported by a pillow. Also called the *dorsal recumbent* position.

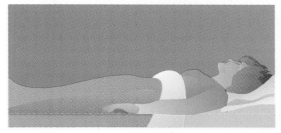

PRONE

- The client lies flat on his or her stomach. The head is supported by a pillow.

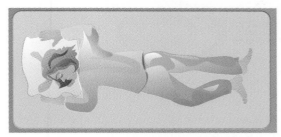

LATERAL RECUMBENT

- The client lies on the side that is indicated. Pillows are positioned to support the head and the higher leg and may be put at the client's back for support. This position is generally not used for elderly clients because of the pressure it puts on their hips.

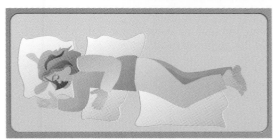

SIMS'

- The shoulders of the client are nearly prone while the hips are in the lateral recumbent position and the upper leg is raised sharply. Pillows support the head, upper arm, and upper leg.

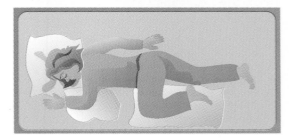

Moving a Client up in Bed

When clients are sitting in bed, it is easy for them to slide down into a position of poor body alignment. When that happens, move the client back up into the correct position. When moving elderly clients, be sure not to slide them against the sheets. This can damage their skin.

1. PREPARATION

- Follow the preparation guidelines on pages 114-115 as indicated by the Preparation Symbol. Pay special attention to the guidelines on *Positioning the Client* on page 158.

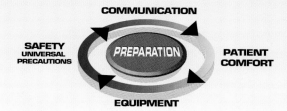

COMMUNICATION

SAFETY
UNIVERSAL
PRECAUTIONS

PREPARATION

PATIENT
COMFORT

EQUIPMENT

- If using a hospital bed, put the bed in the horizontal position at a comfortable height for you to work.
- If using side rails, remove or lower them on the side you will stand. The rail on the far side should be raised for safety.

2. PREPARE CLIENT

- Fan-fold covers to foot of bed. Fan-folds are small multiple folds like those of an accordion.
- Remove all pillows supporting the client and place one against the headboard.

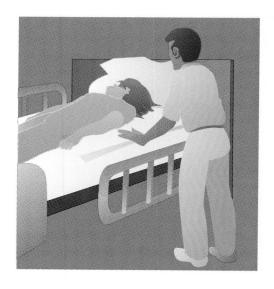

➡ *Make sure not to expose the client.*

MOVING THE CLIENT UP IN BED WITH ASSISTANCE

If a client is too heavy or cannot help, two people can move the client using a procedure similar to the one below. With side rails lowered or removed, two people on either side of the bed lock arms under the client's thighs and shoulders by grasping each other's forearms. They then lift the client forward into position, being careful not to hit the client's head on the headboard.

---

3. POSITION FOR MOVE

- If the clients are able to help, ask them to grab the headboard and put their feet flat on the bed. Ask them to pull with their arms and push with their feet on the count of three.

- Stand across from the client's waist. Your feet should be about one foot apart and the foot closest to the head of the bed should be pointed toward it.

4. MOVE AND COMPLETE

- Place one arm under the client's thighs and the other arm under his or her shoulders.

- **Bend your knees. Keep your back straight.** On the count of three, lift and move smoothly. Step toward the head of the bed.

- Smooth sheets. Replace pillows and covers. Replace side rails, if used.

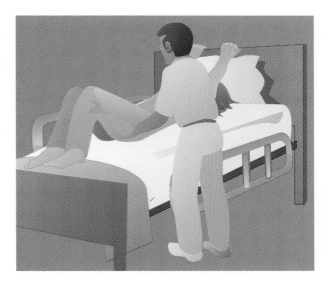

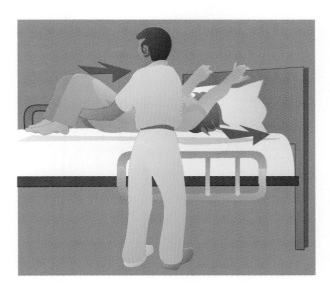

➡ *Remember to speak clearly so the client can understand you.*

Follow the completion guidelines on pages 124-125 as indicated by the Completion Symbol. Pay special attention to the guidelines on *Positioning the Client* on page 158.

Using a Lifting Sheet

A lifting (or turning) sheet is a folded sheet or draw sheet used by **two** people to lift heavy or immobile clients. It places less physical stress on clients since their weight is evenly spread over the sheet. It also keeps the straight body alignment needed for spine and hip disorders.

PROCEDURE

1. PREPARATION

- Follow the preparation guidelines on pages 114-115 as indicated by the Preparation Symbol. Pay special attention to the guidelines on *Positioning the Client* on page 158.

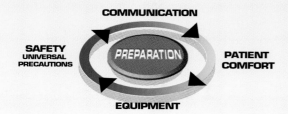

- Get another person to assist you.
- If using a hospital bed, put the bed in the horizontal position at a comfortable height for you to work.
- If using side rails, lower or remove.

2. ROLL SHEET

- Fan-fold covers to foot of bed and pull the edges of the lifting sheet from under the mattress.
- Remove all pillows supporting the client and place one against the headboard.
- With the client in the center of the bed, each lifter rolls up the edges of the sheet to the client's sides.

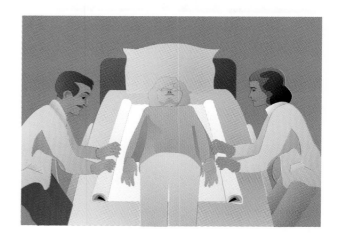

➥ *If a family member is helping you, be sure to carefully explain each step before attempting it. Ask the person to repeat what you have said.*

➥ *Make sure not to expose the client. If necessary, cover the client with a bath blanket.*

POINTERS

162

If there is no turning sheet on the bed, you may place one under the client by:

1) turning the client on his or her side;

2) placing a folded sheet behind and alongside the client;

3) moving the client back over the fold so that you can unfold the sheet.

3. POSITION FOR MOVE

- Ask clients to place their feet flat on the mattress so the weight of their legs is supported when you lift.

- Each lifter stands across from the client's waist. Your feet should be about one foot apart and the foot closest to the head of the bed should be pointed toward it.

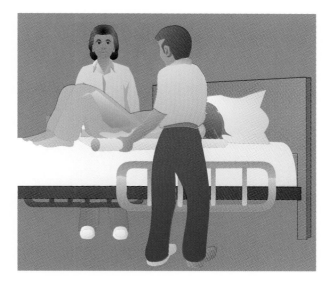

4. MOVE AND COMPLETE

- Grasp the rolled sheet near the client's thighs and shoulders.

- **Bend your knees. Keep your back straight.** On the count of three, both lifters should lift and move smoothly. Step toward the head of the bed.

- Smooth sheets. Replace pillows and covers.

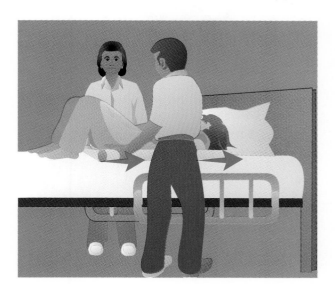

Follow the completion guidelines on pages 124-125 as indicated by the Completion Symbol. Pay special attention to the guidelines on *Positioning the Client* on page 158.

Moving a Client to One Side

Clients are moved to one side of the bed for a number of reasons, including making an occupied bed and for positioning them on their sides. Moving the client by yourself requires moving the client in the steps described below. A lifting sheet may be used when you have assistance.

1. PREPARATION

- Follow the preparation guidelines on pages 114-115 as indicated by the Preparation Symbol. Pay special attention to the guidelines on *Positioning the Client* on page 158.

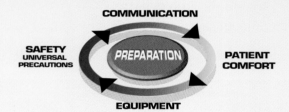

- If using a hospital bed, put the bed in the horizontal position at a comfortable height for you to work.

- If using side rails, remove or lower them on the side you will stand. The rail on the far side should be raised for safety.

- Fan-fold covers to foot of bed and remove all pillows supporting client.

2. MOVE UPPER BODY

- Stand facing the client's shoulders, with one foot slightly back.

- Cross the client's arms over his or her chest. Place one arm under the client's shoulder and the other arm under the client's middle back. Smoothly slide the client toward you while shifting your weight onto your back foot.

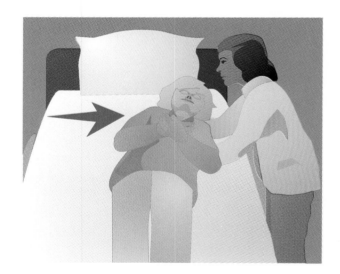

➡ *Make sure not to expose the client.*

➡ *Tell the client when you are going to begin sliding.*

3. MOVE HIPS

- Stand facing the client's hips, with one foot slightly back.
- Place one arm under the client's waist and the other arm under the client's thighs. Smoothly slide the client toward you while shifting your weight onto your back foot.

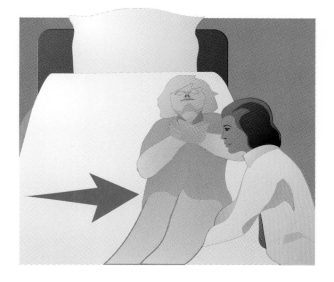

➡ *Be careful not to drag or jerk the client.*

4. MOVE LEGS

- Stand facing the client's knees, with one foot slightly back.
- Place one arm under the client's thighs and the other arm under the client's calves. Smoothly slide the client toward you while shifting your weight onto your back foot. The client should be lined up on the desired side.

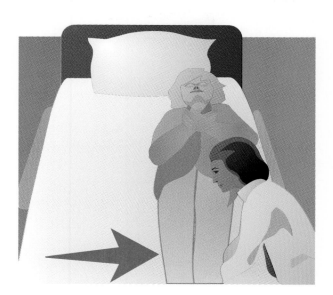

Follow the completion guidelines on pages 124-125 as indicated by the Completion Symbol. Pay special attention to the guidelines on *Positioning the Client* on page 158.

Turning a Client

You will turn clients on their sides for a number of reasons, including making an occupied bed, repositioning during bedrest, and for various procedures. (For clients with spine or hip disorders, the client's body is kept completely straight and rigid during turning. Using a draw sheet will help this. See the procedure on *Logrolling* on page 168.)

See the procedure on *Logrolling* on page 168.

PROCEDURE

1. PREPARATION

- Follow the preparation guidelines on pages 114-115 as indicated by the Preparation Symbol. Pay special attention to the guidelines on *Positioning the Client* on page 158.

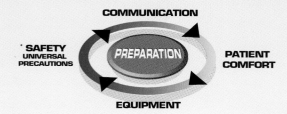

- If using a hospital bed, put the bed in the horizontal position at a comfortable height for you to work.
- If using side rails, remove or lower them on the side you will stand. The rail on the far side should be raised for safety.
- Fan-fold covers to foot of bed and remove all pillows.

2a. TURNING TOWARD

- Stand across from the client's waist, facing the bed, on the side to which you want to turn the client.
- Cross the client's arms over his or her chest and the far leg over the near leg.
- Turn the client on his or her side by gently rolling the client's far shoulder and hip toward you.

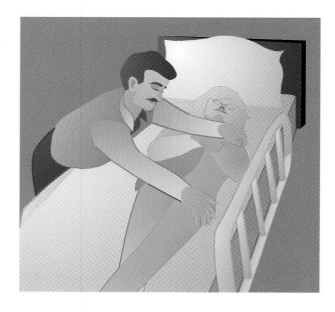

POINTERS

➡ Make sure not to expose the client. Use a bath blanket if necessary.

➡ *If you want clients to finish in the center of the bed, move them to the **far** side of the bed when you begin.*

SIMS' POSITION

If assisting the client into the Sims' position, turn the shoulders of the client to a nearly prone position (see page 159). Help the client to free the lower arm and position the hips in the lateral recumbent position with the upper leg raised sharply. Support the head, upper arm, and upper leg with pillows.

2b. TURNING AWAY

- Stand across from the client's waist, facing the bed, opposite the side to which you will turn the client.
- Cross the client's arms over the chest and the near leg over the far leg.
- Turn the client on his or her side by gently lifting the client's near shoulder and hip.

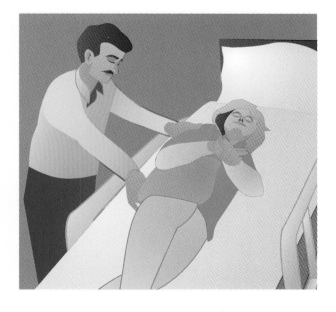

➡ *If you want clients to finish in the center of the bed, move them to the near side of the bed when you begin.*

3. COMPLETION

- Place pillows under the head, upper thigh and leg, and the arm and hand.
- Smooth sheets. Replace covers.

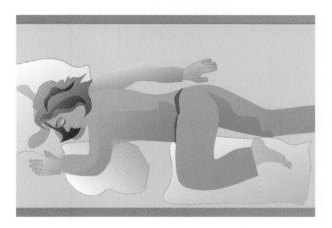

Follow the completion guidelines on pages 124-125 as indicated by the Completion Symbol. Pay special attention to the guidelines on *Positioning the Client* on page 158.

Logrolling

For clients with spine or hip disorders, a draw sheet can be used to keep the client's body completely straight and rigid during turning. Two people use the draw sheet to roll the client in a single motion like a log.

PROCEDURE

1. PREPARATION

- Follow the preparation guidelines on pages 114-115 as indicated by the Preparation Symbol. Pay special attention to the guidelines on *Positioning the Client* on page 158.

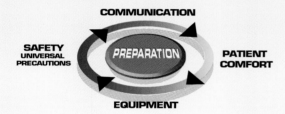

- If using a hospital bed, put the bed in the horizontal position at a comfortable height for you to work.

- If using side rails, remove or lower them on the side you will stand. The rail on the far side should be raised for safety.

- Fan-fold covers to foot of bed and remove all pillows.

➥ *If a family member is helping you, be sure to carefully explain each step before attempting it. Ask the person to repeat what you have said.*

➥ *Make sure not to expose the client. Use a bath blanket if necessary.*

2. MOVE TO SIDE

- Position the client on one side of the bed so he or she will be in the center after being turned. Follow the procedure on Using a Lifting Sheet on pages 162-163 but pull the sheet and client to one side instead of toward the headboard.

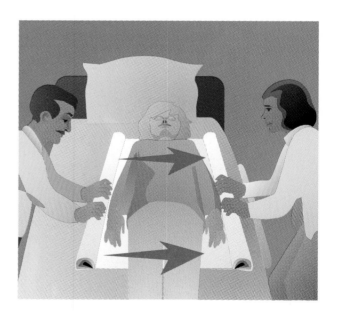

➥ *Ask the client to stiffen his or her body as much as possible. Make sure to keep the client's body straight and rigid while you move the client.*

POINTERS

3. POSITION FOR ROLL

- With the client positioned on the side of the bed, cross the client's arms over his or her chest and **place a pillow lengthwise between the client's legs** from the knees to the ankles.

- If using side rails, replace or raise on that side. Then go to the other side of the bed. One person stands at the client's hips and one stands at the shoulders.

4. ROLL AND COMPLETE

- They grasp the sheet on the far side with both hands at the shoulder and hips and turn the client by gently pulling.

- Smooth sheets. Position pillows (see page 167, step 3) and replace covers.

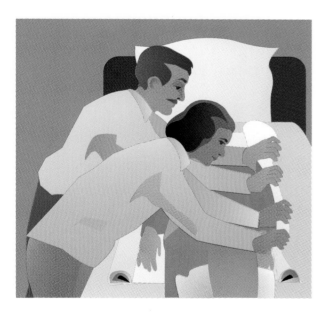

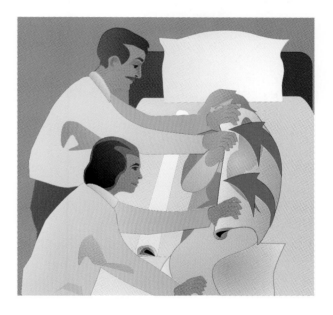

Follow the completion guidelines on pages 124-125 as indicated by the Completion Symbol. Pay special attention to the guidelines on *Positioning the Client* on page 158.

Sitting on the Edge of the Bed

You will help clients to sit at the edge of the bed for many procedures and to prepare them for getting out of bed. Also called **dangling**, clients may be required to swing or dangle their legs from the edge of the bed for a period of time as part of their care.

PROCEDURE

1. PREPARATION

- Follow the preparation guidelines on pages 114-115 as indicated by the Preparation Symbol. Pay special attention to the guidelines on *Positioning the Client* on page 158.

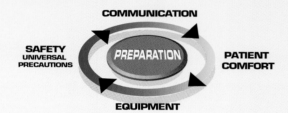

- If using a hospital bed, put the bed in the horizontal position at a comfortable height for you to work.
- If using side rails, remove or lower them on the side you will stand. The rail on the far side should be raised for safety.
- Fan-fold covers to foot of bed and remove all pillows.

➥ *Make sure not to expose the client.*

2. POSITION CLIENT

- Following the procedure on Moving the Client to One Side on pages 126-127, move the client to the side of the bed over which he or she will dangle.
- Bring the client to a sitting position either with pillows or by raising the head of the bed.

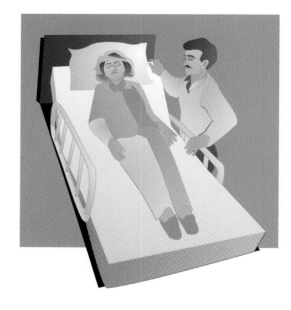

➥ *When clients will be getting out of bed, you may need to help them get dressed.* **Put footwear on while they are still in bed.** *Protect the bedsheet from soiling by placing paper under their feet.*

POINTERS

SPECIAL PRECAUTIONS

Clients sitting on the edge of the bed need close supervision. You may need to support them with a pillow behind the back. If they show any signs of dizziness or unsteadiness, return them to bed by reversing this procedure. Report the problem immediately to your supervisor.

3. CRADLE & TURN

- Cradle the client's knees with one arm and the client's shoulders with the other.
- On the count of three, turn the client in a sitting position so his or her legs move over the edge of the bed.

4. DANGLE

- Support the client until you are sure he or she is steady and composed. Check breathing and pulse.
- If the client is getting out of bed and you are using a hospital bed, lower the bed until the client's feet touch the floor.

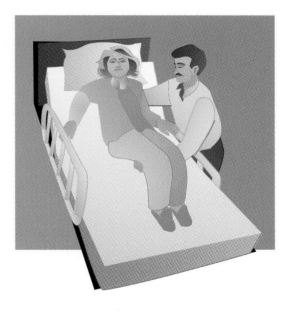

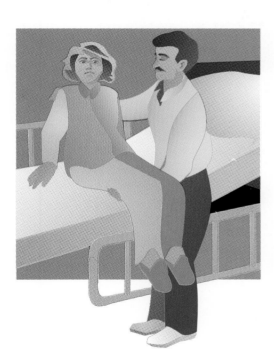

➡ *If clients are capable, ask them to help you on the count of three by pushing up with their arms and swinging their legs over the edge of the bed.*

Follow the completion guidelines on pages 124-125 as indicated by the Completion Symbol. Pay special attention to the guidelines on *Positioning the Client* on page 158.

Positioning a Client in Bed

1.
Imagine yourself as a home care client. How do you think you would feel about an aide touching you, positioning you, or lifting you?

2.
Which of the positions on page 159 do you use when you sleep or rest? If you were awake and undergoing bedrest, how long do you think you would be comfortable in each of those positions?

3.
What do you think your clients should know about positioning in bed?

4.
What do you think are the most important things for home care aides to remember when positioning a client in bed?

REVIEW

**Key Terms – Test your understanding of each of these first.
Then use each one once to fill in the incomplete statements below.**

decubitus

side rails

fowler's position

supine

prone

lateral recumbent

sims

draw sheet

logrolling

dangling

1. Clients positioned on their side are in the _____ position.

2. In _____ , the client is sitting at about a 45 degree angle.

3. A _____ is used by two people to lift or move a heavy or immobile client.

4. In _____ , two home care aides use a draw sheet to roll the client in a single motion.

5. Clients on extensive bedrest are moved and repositioned to prevent the development of _____ ulcers.

6. A similar position to the lateral recumbent is _____ , except that the chest is nearly prone.

7. A client sitting on the edge of the bed is said to be

    _____.

8. Removable or attached _____ are often used as a safety precaution when positioning clients in bed.

9. In the _____ position, the client lies horizontally on their back. The _____ position is the opposite.

Transferring a Client

Home care aides regularly *transfer* (move) clients out of their beds.

They assist clients to walk *(ambulation)*. They help clients to a chair so that they can be out of bed for a while. They transfer clients by wheelchair.

It is important to keep clients from falling when moving them out of bed.

Clients who require assistance to move are at serious risk of falling and receiving injury. They are more likely to suddenly feel faint or dizzy and lose their balance.

Pay special attention to safety precautions.

Make sure you have whatever assistance you need and you are certain you can complete the procedure safely. Use good body mechanics (pages 92-93).

Client cooperation is important.

Clients can often help, making the move safer and easier. More importantly, they can tell you when they are feeling faint, dizzy, uncomfortable, or in pain. This will help you to avoid accidents or injury.

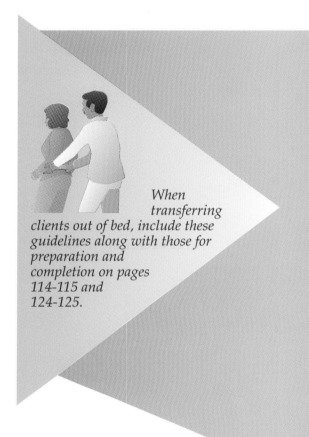

When transferring clients out of bed, include these guidelines along with those for preparation and completion on pages 114-115 and 124-125.

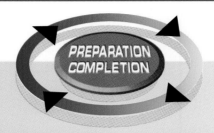

Communication

✔ Speak clearly. Clients need to be able to follow your directions.

✔ Ask clients to tell you any time they don't feel well or are uncomfortable.

✔ Make moves on a count of three.

✔ Check pulse and breathing after moving clients and report results to your supervisor.

Comfort

✔ Make sure clients are appropriately dressed and comfortable with their clothing.

✔ Make sure transfer belts are snug but not tight.

✔ Check clients sitting in chairs or wheelchairs frequently. Reposition clients who are uncomfortable or have moved out of proper position.

✔ Use wheelchair cushions or blankets to prevent uncomfortable perspiration for clients in wheelchairs.

✔ Know if a client has a weak side, and adjust movements for it.

Equipment

✔ Be completely familiar with equipment before you use it. Check manufacturer's instructions and agency guidelines.

✔ Make sure the equipment works before you use it. Check wheelchair brakes to make sure they hold.

Safety

✔ Use safety rails and belts as indicated. Make sure wheelchair brakes are locked.

✔ Position furniture so it will not be in your way when you move the client.

✔ Make sure clients have non-skid footwear whenever they are to stand or walk.

✔ Be alert for fainting or dizziness. Return any client feeling faint or dizzy to bed immediately and tell your supervisor.

Moving to a Chair

The procedure for moving clients to a chair or wheelchair is the same except that the wheels of the wheelchair are locked and the client's feet are placed on footrests. **Clients in chairs or wheelchairs need to be frequently checked and repositioned.** To move the client from a chair to bed, the procedure is reversed.

PROCEDURE

1. PREPARATION

- Follow the preparation guidelines on pages 114-115 as indicated by the Preparation Symbol. Pay special attention to the guidelines on *Transferring a Client* on page 175.

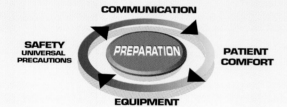

- Position the chair or wheelchair next to the bed. **Lock the wheels on a wheelchair.**

- Position the client on the edge of the bed. Help the client put on clothes. Put non-skid footwear and a safety belt (if indicated) on the client.

- Make sure the client is steady and relaxed and his or her feet are on the floor.

⇒ *If the client is faint or dizzy, return him or her to bed and tell your supervisor.*

⇒ *If the client has a weak side, place the chair on the opposite side of the bed so the strong side will lead through the move.*

2. POSITION FOR LIFT

- Face the client with your hips and shoulders squared and your feet about a foot apart, blocking the client's feet.

- Bending at the knees, lower yourself and grasp the safety belt on each side of client's waist (or reach under the client's arms and grasp the client's upper back).

- Place your knees against the client's.

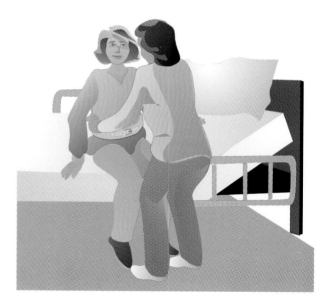

⇒ *Positioning your knees and feet around the client's will protect the client from slipping.*

POINTERS

Safety belts (also called *transfer* or *gait* belts) allow you to lift or steady clients during moving by grasping the belt. They are applied around the waist over the client's clothing. Follow the manufacturer's directions for using the belt. Make sure it is secure enough to stay in position but never tight enough to chafe or cut off circulation.

3. STAND AND TURN

- Ask the client to stand on the count of three. The client should lean forward to maintain balance and push off the bed with his or her arms. On count of three, raise to an erect position, gently lifting the client with you.
- Slowly turn with the client until you are facing the chair and the client is directly in front of it.

4. LOWER TO CHAIR

- Ask the client to sit on the count of three. Gently lower the client by bending at the knees.
- Position the client comfortably with the back straight and buttocks completely to the rear of the chair. When using a wheelchair, place the client's feet on the footrests. Remove safety belt.

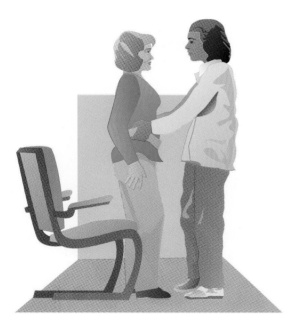

➡ *The chair seat should touch the back of the client's legs and the arms of the chair should be within the client's reach.*

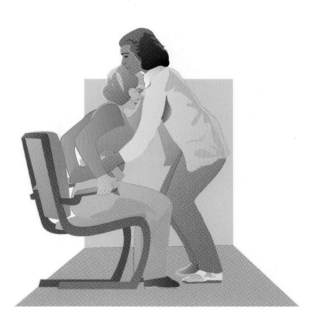

Follow the completion guidelines on pages 124-125 as indicated by the Completion Symbol. Pay special attention to the guidelines on *Transferring a Client* on page 175.

Moving a Non-ambulatory Client

To move *non-ambulatory* clients (clients who cannot walk) to a wheelchair requires at least two people. In many cases a *mechanical lift* will be used (pages 180-181). Clients being moved by wheelchair must always be appropriately clothed and covered and never left alone.

(pages 180-181)

PROCEDURE

1. PREPARATION

- Follow the preparation guidelines on pages 114-115 as indicated by the Preparation Symbol. Pay special attention to the guidelines on *Transferring a Client* on page 175.

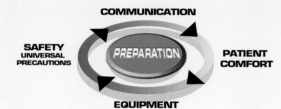

COMMUNICATION

SAFETY UNIVERSAL PRECAUTIONS

PREPARATION

PATIENT COMFORT

EQUIPMENT

- Position the client on one side of the bed following the guidelines on pages 164-165. Help the client put on clothes and footwear.
- Raise the client to a sitting position by raising the head of the bed. One person supports the client in this position.

EQUIPMENT

- Wheelchair with armrests that can be removed.

➡ *Check with your supervisor to see under what circumstances you may perform this procedure.*

2. POSITION CLIENT AND CHAIR

- Ask the client to lock arms across the stomach.
- Position the wheelchair across from the client's hips, facing the foot of the bed.
- Remove the wheelchair armrest closest to the bed and lock the wheels. Place a cushion on the seat if indicated.

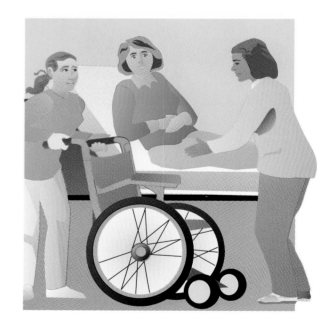

➡ *Wheelchair cushions are sometimes necessary for clients to prevent perspiration against the vinyl.*

POINTERS

3. CRADLE CLIENT

- One person stands behind the wheelchair by the client's shoulders and one stands before it facing the client's thighs.

- The person by the client's shoulders reaches under the client's arms from behind and locks arms in front of the client's chest. The other person cradles the client's thighs and calves.

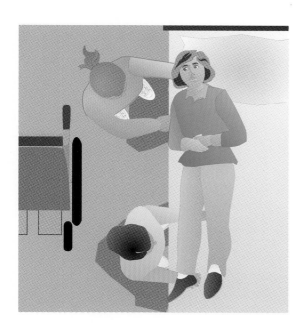

➡ *Remember to bend your knees and keep your back straight.*

4. LIFT AND MOVE

- On the count of three, the person at the client's shoulders raises to a standing position, lifting the client over the back of the wheelchair. At the same time, the other person lifts the client's legs and lowers the client's buttocks to the rear of the chair.

- Make sure the client is comfortable and his or her back is straight. Place the client's feet on the footrests.

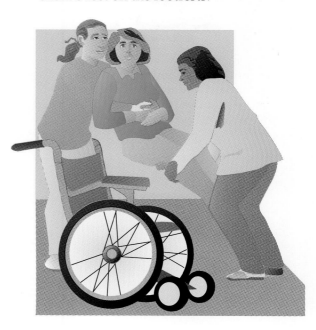

Follow the completion guidelines on pages 124-125 as indicated by the Completion Symbol. Pay special attention to the guidelines on *Transferring a Client* on page 175.

Using a Mechanical Lift

Mechanical lifts are used to lift clients who either cannot move or have difficulty moving to and from beds, wheelchairs, and bathtubs. Ideally, one person operates the lift while another guides the client down — as we show in the procedure below. However, many transfers with a mechanical lift can be performed safely by a single home care aide. **If you have to use a mechanical lift, follow the manufacturer's instructions and pay close attention to safety.** The procedure is reversed to return the client to bed.

PROCEDURE

1. PREPARATION

- Follow the preparation guidelines on pages 114-115 as indicated by the Preparation Symbol. Pay special attention to the guidelines on *Transferring a Client* on page 175.

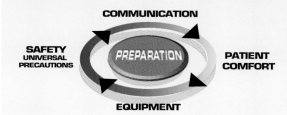

- **Be completely familiar with the equipment and make sure it works before you use it.** Check manufacturer's instructions and agency guidelines.
- Clothe the client appropriately.

EQUIPMENT

- Mechanical lift with instructions.
- Wheelchair.

2. POSITION SLING

- Position the sling underneath the client by turning the client from side to side (see pages 166-167) over the folded sling. One person can support the client while the other positions the sling along the client's back.
- Center the client on the sling in the supine position with arms crossed over the chest.

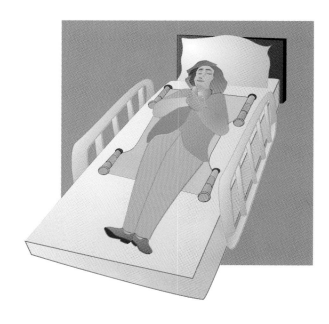

➧ *Make sure the sling is positioned according to the manufacturer's instructions.*

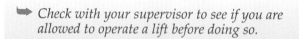

➧ *Check with your supervisor to see if you are allowed to operate a lift before doing so.*

POINTERS

3. POSITION LIFT

- Position the lift at the side of the bed and center the boom over the client. **Lock the lift's wheels.**

- Attach the chains to the sling and swivel bar, with the **open ends of the S-hooks pointed away from the client.**

- One person uses the lift to raise the client off the bed while the other guides the client.

4. MOVE CLIENT

- Unlock wheels and move the lift and client away from the bed to position the client over the wheelchair. **Lock wheels of lift and chair.**

- One person gently lowers the client while the other guides him or her into the chair. Unhook the sling but leave it in place for reversing the procedure.

- Make sure the client is comfortable and positioned in good body alignment.

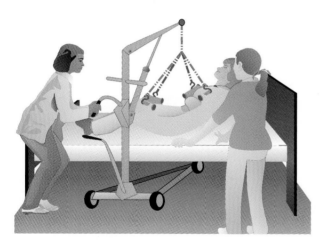

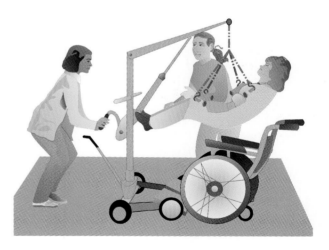

Follow the completion guidelines on pages 124-125 as indicated by the Completion Symbol. Pay special attention to the guidelines on *Transferring a Client* on page 175.

➡ *Chains should be same length on each side of client.*

Assisted Walking

Assisting clients to walk is a common activity for home care aides. You will sometimes use a safety *(transfer or gait)* belt to reduce the risk of falling. You will also use a technique for supporting falling clients that will lessen injuries. Begin by assisting the client to a standing position, following the guidelines for *Moving to a Chair* on pages 176-177. Return the client to bed by reversing the procedure.

PROCEDURE

USING A SAFETY BELT

- Stand slightly behind and to the side of the client on the client's weak side.
- Grasp the safety belt behind the client with your hand closest the client using an underhand grip. With your other hand, grasp the side of the belt or the client's hand.
- Walk slowly on same foot with the client.

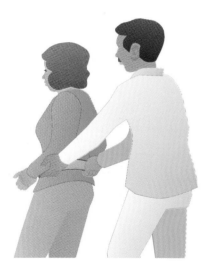

- ➠ *The illustration shows the home care aide grasping the safety belt and moving into position. When walking, he will be closer to the client's side.*
- ➠ *Standing on the client's weak side will allow you to provide more support.*

BREAKING A FALL

- At the start of a fall, pull the client toward you and support him or her under the arms.
- Bring your outside leg back a step for support and gently slide the client down your angled front leg.
- Check that the client is alright. Follow your agency's policy for checking vital signs, getting help, and for returning the client to bed.

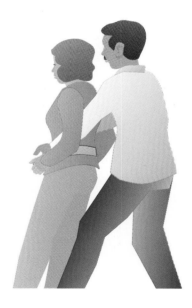

- ➠ *Your agency will have strict guidelines on how to handle client falls. Know the policy and follow it. You will have to file an incident report.*

POINTERS

USING A CANE

- A cane is always held at hip level on the client's strong side (for support). It is placed about six inches to the side and twelve inches in front of the foot.
- The weak leg is brought forward even with the cane (#1).
- Then the strong leg steps ahead of both (#2). This is repeated by bringing the cane 12 inches forward and continuing the steps.

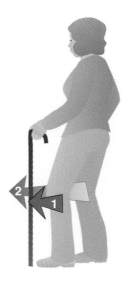

➡ *Check the rubber tip of the cane to see that it is in good condition.*

➡ *The height of the cane should cause the client's arm to bend slightly while supporting on the cane and allow an erect posture while walking.*

USING A WALKER

- The client holds on to both sides of the walker. With feet spread about six inches apart for balance, the walker is lifted and moved six inches forward.
- One foot is brought forward six inches, and then the other is. The feet are spread apart for balance. The action is repeated by bringing the walker forward six inches and continuing the steps.

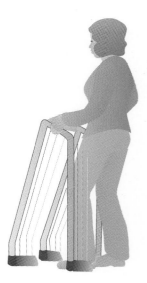

➡ *Check the rubber tips of the walker to see that they are in good condition.*

➡ *The height of the walker should cause the client's arms to bend slightly while supporting on the walker and allow an erect posture while walking.*

Transferring a Client

1.
Remember a few times that you fell. Why did they happen?

2.
If you were a client that needed assistance to move out of bed, how would you want home care aides to act when helping you?

3.
What do you think a client should know about movement out of bed?

4.
What do you think are the most important things to remember when assisting clients to move out of bed?

REVIEW

**Key Terms – Test your understanding of each of these first.
Then use each one once to fill in the incomplete statements below.**

pulse and breathing

strong side

non-skid footwear

brakes

safety belt

mechanical lift

cane

walker

incident report

1. _____ must be worn by the client when getting out of bed.

2. The client always holds a _____ on his or her strong side for support.

3. When clients fall, you will have to file an _____ _____.

4. You should always check the client's _____ after transferring him or her out of bed.

5. _____ must always be applied to wheelchair, bed, and mechanical lift wheels as a safety precaution during moves.

6. A _____ (also called a transfer or gait belt) allows you to lift or steady clients during moving or walking by grasping the belt, not the client or their clothing.

7. A _____ is moved forward six inches at a time and the client then steps up to it.

8. When helping a client out of bed, lead with their _____ .

9. A _____ is used to lift immobile clients to and from beds, wheelchairs, and bathtubs.

Personal Care

Personal care is important for health and self-esteem.

Personal care includes all the activities of *personal hygiene* (keeping yourself clean) and *grooming* (keeping a neat appearance). These areas directly affect how we feel about ourselves and how others see us.

Home care aides regularly assist clients to perform personal care.

Many clients will not be able to perform personal care without assistance. You will help clients to bathe, brush teeth, shave, dress, etc. You will also give back massages to ensure healthy skin.

Providing personal care will put you in close physical contact with clients.

You must be very sensitive to the client's comfort and personal dignity, and to safety risks (infection, falling, etc.) to both the client and yourself.

Personal care is a form of self-expression.

Most people have developed habits in performing their own personal care. You must accept and respect these habits. You must also help clients towards the goal of caring for themselves: the more of their own personal care they provide, the better they will feel about themselves.

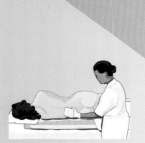

When providing personal care, include these guidelines along with those for preparation and completion on pages 114-115 and 124-125.

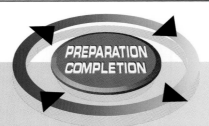

PREPARATION
COMPLETION

Communication

✔ Speak clearly. The client needs to be able to follow your directions.

✔ Remember that hygiene and grooming are personal activities. Ask clients how they would like you to assist them. Do as they ask whenever you can.

✔ Encourage the client to perform as much self-care as possible.

✔ Observe and report any unusual physical or emotional changes.

Client Comfort

✔ Be sure to maintain the client's privacy and not expose them during bathing, dressing, etc.

✔ Use special care in providing or assisting in oral hygiene. The mouth, gums, and teeth can be very sensitive. So can the client's feelings.

✔ Use skin lotions (approved by your agency) to keep clients' skin from drying or chapping.

Equipment

✔ Clients' personal care items (toothbrush, comb, clothing, etc.) are personal property. Handle them with care.

Safety

✔ Use a bath thermometer to check water temperature for washing and bathing. Make sure the temperature is kept to 105-110 degrees.

✔ Be alert. Wet floors are dangerous.

✔ Never leave a client who needs assistance alone in a tub or shower.

✔ Follow *Universal Precautions* any time there is a possibility of contact with blood or body fluids (feces, urine, vomitus, etc.).

✔ Pay close attention to the condition of the client's skin and be alert for any reddened, discolored, or swollen areas. Be sure to provide preventative skin care.

Brushing Teeth

Brushing teeth is usually performed at the start and end of the day and after meals. Clients should be encouraged to do their own brushing, but at times you will need to assist. The procedure below is for brushing a client's teeth while the client remains in bed or a chair. Because of the close physical contact this requires, you must be considerate and sensitive to the client's feelings. **You must also practice Universal Precautions because of the possibility of coming in contact with the client's blood from bleeding gums or other causes.**

PROCEDURE

1. PREPARATION

- Follow the preparation guidelines on pages 114-115 as indicated by the Preparation Symbol. Pay special attention to the guidelines on *Personal Care* on page 187.

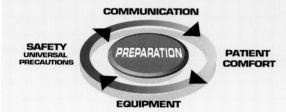

- Place your equipment on top of a paper towel on a surface convenient for you to work.

EQUIPMENT

- paper towels
- face towel
- disposable gloves
- toothbrush
- toothpaste
- cup with water
- small basin
- dental floss
- cup of mouthwash
- tissues

➡ *If you don't have a small basin, any wide mouth cup or glass will do.*

2. POSITION CLIENT

- Raise the client to a sitting position. If using side rails, remove or lower the rail on the side you will stand.
- Place the face towel over the client's chest below his or her chin. **Put on disposable gloves.**

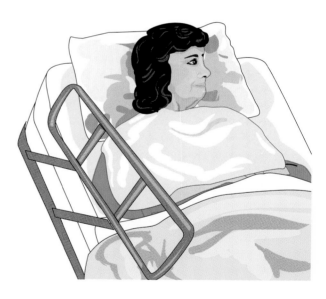

➡ *If clients cannot be raised to a sitting position, place them in the side-lying position.*

➡ *Ask clients if they have any sore areas in their mouths or any preferences about brushing. Take their answers into consideration when you brush.*

POINTERS

ORAL HYGIENE

Cavities, gum disease, infections, and bad breath are among the many problems that result from poor oral hygiene. To prevent this, you will assist clients to brush and floss their teeth and take care of their dentures. You will also help and encourage them towards self-care. As you assist in oral hygiene, pay close attention to the condition of the client's teeth, gums, and mouth, and report any problems you see to your supervisor.

3. BRUSH TEETH

- Put toothpaste on the brush and wet it by pouring water onto it over the basin.
- Gently brush the inside and outside of the teeth with a horizontal back-and-forth motion. For the inside of the front teeth, hold the brush at an angle and use a side to side motion.

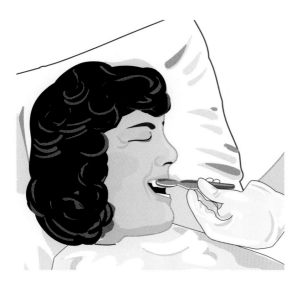

➡ *Be careful not to put the brush far enough into the mouth to cause choking.*

➡ *Be alert to the condition of the mouth. Note any sores, bleeding, or discoloration and report them to your supervisor.*

4. RINSE AND COMPLETE

- Give the client water to rinse. Hold the basin under the client's chin so he or she can spit into the basin. Wipe the client's mouth if needed.
- Floss teeth if it is ordered (see page 190). Have client rinse with mouthwash if ordered or desired.

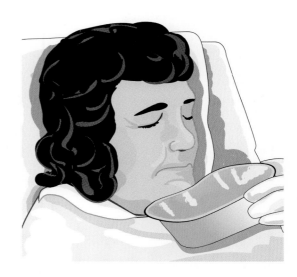

Follow the completion guidelines on pages 124-125 as indicated by the Completion Symbol. Pay special attention to the guidelines on *Personal Care* on page 187.

Flossing Teeth

Flossing teeth removes tartar and food particles from surfaces difficult to clean with a toothbrush. Besides cleaning teeth, flossing helps maintain healthy gums and should generally be performed at least once a day after the last meal. Flossing may cause the gums to bleed, however, and will not always be ordered. Only floss when it is ordered. **Follow regular preparation and completion guidelines and practice Universal Precautions.**

PROCEDURE

1. HOLDING FLOSS

- **Put on disposable gloves.**
- Take about 18 inches of dental floss and wrap the ends snugly around the middle finger of each hand. Continue winding it around one finger until the fingers are about 8 inches apart.
- Use your thumbs and index fingers to position the floss between the teeth.

2. FLOSSING TEETH

- Gently rub off food particles and plaque from the surfaces between the teeth by moving the floss up and down against the teeth.
- Unwind new floss as needed (generally after every other tooth) while winding the used floss around your other finger.
- Let the client rinse his or her mouth. Dispose of the floss and gloves.

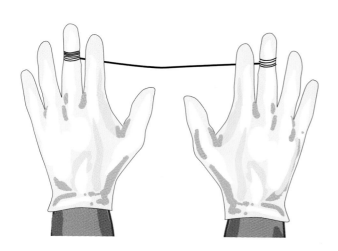

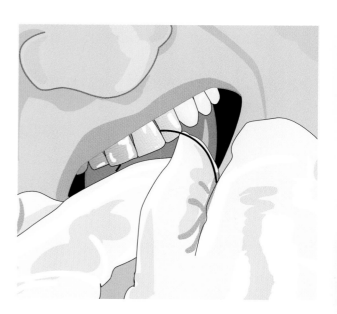

➡ *Only floss if it is ordered.*
➡ *Don't wrap the floss too tightly around your fingers or you will cut off circulation.*

➡ *You can floss under a bridge (see p.192) if you thread the floss between the teeth using a floss threader.*

POINTERS

Oral Care for the Unconscious Client

Personal Care | Unit **14**

The unconscious client's mouth is cleaned every two hours as part of routine care. This keeps the client from breathing in fluid *(aspirating)*, a serious danger. You position the client on his or her side and hold the mouth open and tongue in place with a gauze wrapped tongue blade. You then use special applicators and a cleaning solution to wipe the mouth clean. **Follow regular preparation and completion guidelines and practice Universal Precautions.**

1. POSITION CLIENT

- Tell the client what you will be doing. Position the client on his or her side. Place a towel under the client's head.

- **Put on disposable gloves.** Place a small basin under the chin.

- Open the client's mouth with a tongue blade wrapped in gauze. Use it to hold the mouth open and the tongue in place while you clean with your other hand.

2. WIPE WITH APPLICATORS

- Dip applicators in the cleaning solution used by your agency. Gently wipe the teeth, gums, tongue, and inside surfaces of the mouth with the applicators. Change applicators frequently.

- Rinse the client's mouth with applicators dipped in water.

- Apply petroleum jelly to the lips to keep them from chapping or splitting. Continue with other care.

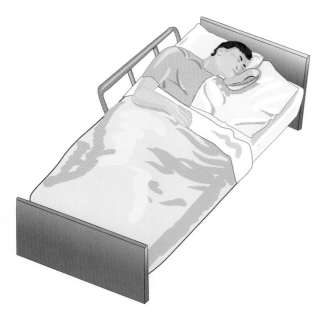

➡ *Remember that **the unconscious client may be able to hear you.** Speak to the client as if he or she can hear you.*

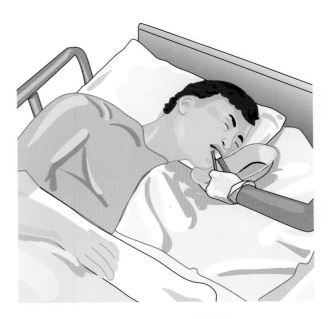

➡ *You may also be directed to wipe the client's mouth with lemon glycerine swabs before applying petroleum jelly to the lips.*

Dentures

Dentures are false teeth that are form-fitted to the gums. They must be cleaned as often as natural teeth. They may be for the whole mouth or a *bridge* of one or more false teeth. They are costly to replace and must be handled carefully to prevent damage and keep their shape. After dentures are removed for cleaning, oral care is given to the client before the dentures are returned to the mouth. **Universal Precautions are used when cleaning dentures.**

PROCEDURE

1. PREPARATION

- Follow the preparation guidelines on pages 114-115 as indicated by the Preparation Symbol. Pay special attention to the guidelines on *Personal Care* on page 187.

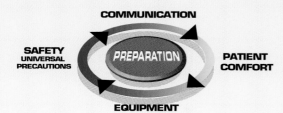

COMMUNICATION

SAFETY
UNIVERSAL
PRECAUTIONS

PREPARATION

PATIENT
COMFORT

EQUIPMENT

- Assemble your equipment, position the client, and put on disposable gloves as in step 2 of *Brushing Teeth* on page 188.

EQUIPMENT

- paper towels
- two face towels
- disposable gloves
- gauze squares
- toothbrush
- cleaner or toothpaste
- cup with water
- small basin
- cup of mouthwash
- tissues
- denture cup

➡ *You must always practice **Universal Precautions** when you provide denture care as you will be exposed to saliva that may contain the client's blood.*

2. REMOVE DENTURES

- Using a gauze pad, grasp the front of the upper denture with your thumb and index finger and loosen the seal by gently moving up and down.
- Carefully pull the upper denture down from the gums and out of the mouth and put in the basin.
- Grasp the lower denture and gently loosen. Lift up and out and put in the basin. Take the basin to a sink.

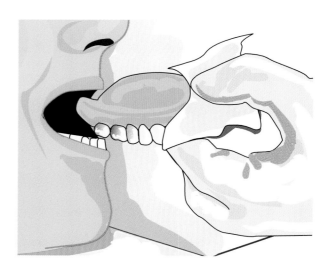

➡ *Allow and encourage the client to take the dentures out and otherwise perform as much oral care as he or she can.*

➡ *Using gauze gives you a better grip on the denture.*

POINTERS

192

3. CLEAN

- Rinse the dentures under warm water and put in the denture cup.
- Line the sink with a face towel and fill it half-way with cool water.
- Apply denture cleaner to the toothbrush. Hold the dentures over the sink and brush them back and forth on the outside first and then up and down on the inside.
- Rinse under warm water, put in the denture cup. Fill it with cool water.

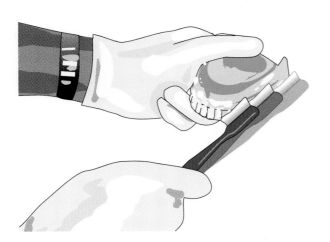

➡ *Never use hot water on dentures. It can warp them.*

➡ *Never store dentures in any other container than the client's denture cup, or they may be mishandled or thrown away by accident. Put the cup within easy reach of the client.*

4. INSERT AND COMPLETE

- Brush client's natural teeth as directed on pages 188-189 and rinse with a mouthwash. Then insert upper dentures while gently lifting the upper lip with the index finger of your free hand. Insert the lower dentures while gently lowering the lower lip.

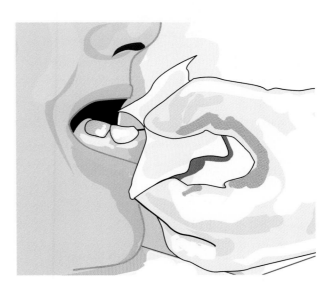

Follow the completion guidelines on pages 124-125 as indicated by the Completion Symbol. Pay special attention to the guidelines on Personal Care on page 187.

COMPLETION

Bed Bath

Bed baths are given to clients who must stay in bed. During it, the client's entire body is washed one part at a time. This requires special sensitivity to the client's privacy and personal dignity. It is a good time to talk with clients and to closely observe their condition. The bed bath is usually performed after elimination and along with oral hygiene and a linen change, though times and frequency will vary by client and care plan.

PROCEDURE

1. PREPARATION

- Follow the preparation guidelines on pages 114-115 as indicated by the Preparation Symbol. Pay special attention to the guidelines on *Personal Care* on page 187.

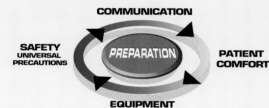

- Place the client in the supine position and cover with a bath blanket. Remove the top linens as in Step 2 on page 152. Remove the client's pajamas or gown (see p.208-209).
- Fill wash basin with warm water (110 degrees), checking with the bath thermometer. Assemble equipment on a surface you will be able to reach.

EQUIPMENT

- wash basin
- soap in soap dish
- nail file or orange stick
- bath thermometer
- washcloths
- bath towels
- paper towels
- bath blanket
- laundry bag
- plastic trash bag
- toilet articles as requested (deodorant, lotion, etc.)
- disposable gloves

2. MAKE A MITT

- **Put on disposable gloves.** Cover the client's chest area with a bath towel.
- Grasp the washcloth between the thumb and knuckle of the index finger of your washing hand.
- Wrap it snugly across your palm and around your four fingers.
- Fold the extra material into your palm and tuck under the bottom edge of the washcloth to form a mitt.

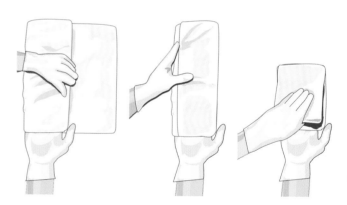

➡ *Make sure the bath blanket covers the client and you do not expose him or her.*

➡ *When wiping the face, make the mitt on your hand closest to the client's hips as you face the client.*

POINTERS

ABOUT THE PROCEDURE

If you are performing a bed bath after helping a client with elimination, you must use a clean new pair of gloves for the bed bath. **After helping the client eliminate, throw away the used gloves, wash your hands, and put on the new gloves.**

3. WASH FACE, NECK, EARS

- Wet the mitt in the basin and squeeze off excess water. Don't use soap unless requested. Using a corner of the mitt, **gently wipe one eye from the inside out.** With the other corner of the mitt, wipe the other eye.

- Wet and soap the mitt. Wipe the face, neck, ears, and behind the ears.

- Rinse the mitt in the basin and then wipe the client with the rinsed mitt. Pat areas dry.

➡ *Wiping each eye with a **different** corner of the mitt prevents the spread of infection from one eye to the other.*

➡ *Always pat rather than rub with the towel to avoid irritating the skin.*

4. ARMS AND SHOULDERS

- Place a bath towel under the client's far arm. Wet and soap the mitt.

- Wash the arm, shoulder, and underarm, while supporting the client's elbow with your free hand.

- Rinse. Pat the arm dry using the towel that is under the arm.

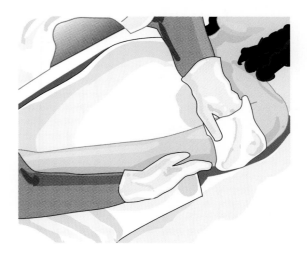

➡ *When washing the arms, the mitt will be on the hand closest to the client's shoulder, while the other hand is used to support the client's arm.*

Bed Bath (Cont'd)

> ### PERSONAL TOILET
>
> Clients often have specific needs and desires on the use of soaps, bath oils, deodorants, anti-perspirants, lotions, powders, etc. You should try to give them what they want as often as possible. However, the use of toilet articles should be watched since they may irritate the skin and are not allowed with certain clients.

PROCEDURE

5. HANDS AND FINGERNAILS

- Position the basin on the bed with the client's hand in the water. Using the mitt and soap, wipe both sides and between the fingers of the hand and rinse in the water.
- Carefully clean under the fingernails with the file or stick (see p.205). Remove the basin and pat dry the hand. Cover arm with bath blanket
- Repeat for the near arm and hand.

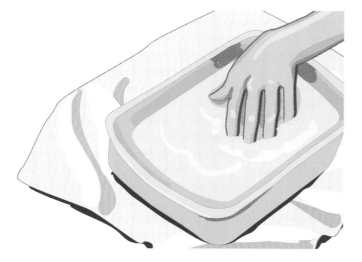

➡ *Replace soapy water with fresh water whenever it becomes cool or cloudy, Make sure the client is safe, covered, and comfortable any time you leave the bedside to get fresh water.*

6. CHEST

- Place a bath towel across the chest. Pull back the bath blanket to the bottom of the towel.
- Lift the towel to wash the chest with the mitt and soap. Rinse and pat dry. On females, be sure to wash, rinse, and dry **under** the breast.
- Turn the towel lengthwise down the chest and abdomen. Pull back the bath blanket to the pubic area. Wash, rinse, and pat dry the abdomen. Pull up the blanket and remove the towel.

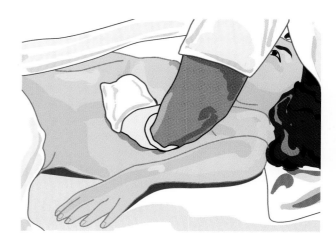

➡ *Make sure you cover the client as much as possible.*
➡ *Keep a dry towel under the part being washed.*

POINTERS

PARTIAL BED BATH

In a partial bed bath, clients wash those areas they can easily reach. You can collect all the equipment necessary for the client and leave while he or she begins. Upon returning, you will generally wash the back, buttocks, underarms, and genitals along with any unwashed areas.

7. LEGS AND FEET

- Place a bath towel under the client's far leg. Lift and support the leg under the knee with your free hand. Then wash the leg with the mitt and soap. Rinse and pat dry.
- Wash the client's foot in the basin as you washed the hand in step 5. Be careful to wash, rinse, and dry between the client's toes. When finished, cover the leg with a bath blanket.
- Repeat for the near leg and foot.

8. BACK AND BUTTOCKS

- Change the bath water.
- Turn client on side to face away from you. Roll up the bath blanket to uncover the back and buttocks and place a bath towel on the bed alongside the back.
- Wash, rinse, and dry from the neck to the buttocks. Cover with the bath blanket.

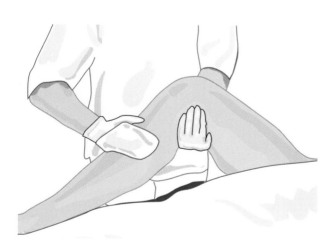

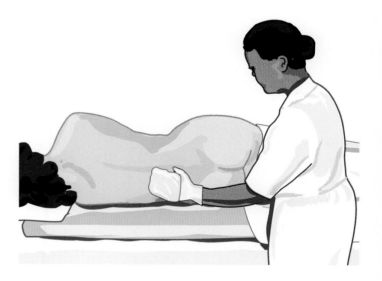

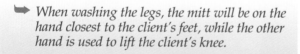

➡ *When washing the legs, the mitt will be on the hand closest to the client's feet, while the other hand is used to lift the client's knee.*

➡ *Provide perineal care following the procedure on pages 198-199.*

Perineal Care

Perineal care (pericare) means cleaning the genitals, anus, and the area between (the *perineum*). It is often performed as part of bathing or any time the area is contaminated by elimination. **This is the most private area of a client's body.** Be very sensitive to the client's sense of privacy and personal dignity when performing pericare. **Use Universal Precautions and encourage self-care.**

PROCEDURE

1. PREPARATION

- **Refill the wash basin with clean, warm (105-110 degrees) water.** Put the washcloths you will use into the water.

- Place the waterproof pad under the client's hips. Spread the client's legs and lift the knees up so the feet are flat on the bed.

- Uncover the perineal area by lifting the bath blanket back toward the abdomen. Wring out a washcloth and make a mitt. Apply soap.

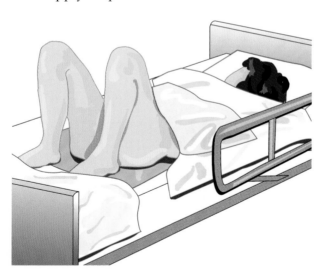

➡ *Be sure you are wearing disposable gloves.*

➡ *A squeeze bottle with warm water or a cleaning solution may be used to wash the perineal area. If so, it is used over a bedpan or toilet.*

2a. FEMALE GENITALS

- Spread the labia with your free hand and **wipe each side of the perineum from the urethral opening *(meatus)* toward the anus in one motion.** Use one side of the mitt and then the other, making sure you are **always wiping with clean cloth.** Replace the washcloth when it is contaminated.

- Repeat until the area is clean.

- Rinse in the same way with a clean cloth. Pat dry.

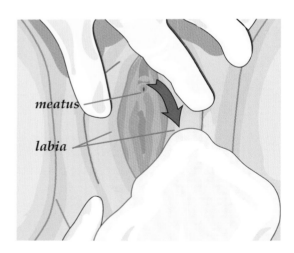

meatus

labia

➡ *Because of the closeness of the anus to the vagina, it is easy to spread fecal bacteria to it. Using a clean cloth and wiping **from top to bottom in one motion** (green arrow) prevents this.*

POINTERS

ABOUT THE PROCEDURE

- The procedure below assumes a continuation of the bed bath from page 197. In addition to the equipment listed on page 194, you will need a waterproof pad.

- If you are providing pericare at another time, assemble the necessary equipment and position the client as indicated in Steps 1 and 2 of the *Bed Bath*.

- If you are assisting in self-care, assemble the equipment for easy use by the client and provide privacy.

2b. MALE GENITALS

- Lift the penis and wipe around the tip (meatus) in a circular motion. Rinse with a clean cloth.

- Wash the rest of the penis by wiping from the tip of the penis to the base. Rinse.

- Wash and rinse each side of the scrotum and the inside of the thighs in the same way. Pat all areas dry.

3. ANAL AREA

- Assist the client to lower his or her legs to the bed and turn to the side-lying position, facing the far side of the bed.

- **Wipe the anal area from the genitals back in one motion.** Wipe first with toilet paper. Then wash the anus one side at a time, using only clean areas of the mitt. Replace the washcloth when it is contaminated.

- Rinse in the same way and pat dry. Remove the waterproof pad and finish by following the guidelines on pages 124-125 and 187.

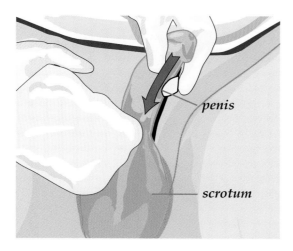

penis

scrotum

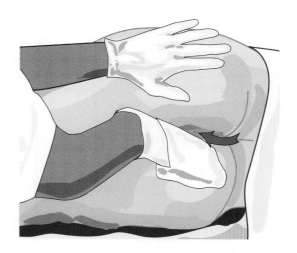

➡ *If the client is not circumcised, pull the foreskin back so you can see the tip of the penis. Then wash the tip and all skin folds.*

➡ *Bacteria from the anus can cause infections if spread to the genital area. You must **always wipe away from the genitals when wiping the anal area.***

COMPLETION

Tub Baths and Showers

You will often assist clients with tub baths and showers in which they perform a large part of the care. While clients may have a greater sense of control and personal dignity than in a bed bath, you must still be very sensitive to their privacy and feelings. **You must also be alert to dangerous situations such as slippery floors, overly hot water, or temporary dizziness.** Also, be careful to avoid drafts.

The steps for a tub bath and a shower are similar. The procedure below is for a tub bath with comments in the *Pointers* highlighting the different steps taken with a shower.

PROCEDURE

1. PREPARATION

- Follow the preparation guidelines on pages 114-115 as indicated by the Preparation Symbol. Pay special attention to the guidelines on *Personal Care* on page 187.

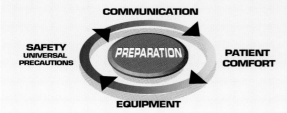

- Assemble equipment near the tub on a handy and clean surface. Use a chair if necessary. Clean the tub with disinfectant if indicated.
- Assist the client from his or her bed to a chair by the tub.

EQUIPMENT

- washcloth
- bath towels
- soap
- bath thermometer
- bath mat
- gown or clothing
- personal toilet articles
- shower chair if necessary

2. FILL THE TUB

- Fill the tub half-way with 105-110 degree water. **Check water temperature with a bath thermometer.**
- Line the bottom of the tub with a towel. Put a bath mat in front of the tub.
- Help the client remove his or her robe, gown, and footwear.

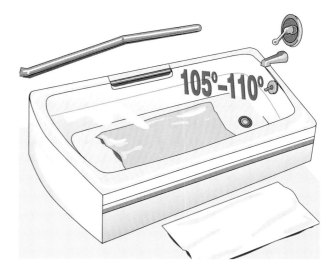

➡ *If the client is taking a shower, place a rubber mat on the shower floor before turning on and adjusting the water temperature.*

➡ *If the client is taking a shower, clean the floor of the shower.*

POINTERS

SOAKS & SITZ BATHS

Soaks — placing parts of the body in water — are often used to apply warmth to the body and as a gentle way to wash it. A *sitz bath* is a type of soak used to wash the perineal area. It is similar to a regular bath, except that the client will just soak the perineal area and hips. The water temperature for a sitz bath is generally around 100-104 degrees, but will be indicated by your nursing supervisor or the client's physician. **Your state may not allow home care aides to administer soaks and sitz baths.** Know your agency and state policies regarding this and follow them.

3. ASSIST THE CLIENT

- Slowly and carefully assist the client into the tub. Ask the client to grasp the safety bar as he or she steps in.
- Let the client wash as much as possible. Wash any areas he or she is unable to reach, such as the back.

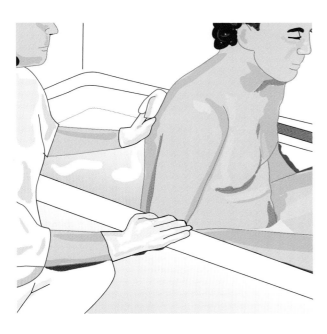

➡ *If the client is taking a shower, be alert to anything that could cause the client to fall: loss of balance, dizziness, etc.*

➡ *You should not leave a client alone in a bath or shower unless your supervisor tells you it is safe to do so.*

4. COMPLETION

- When the client has bathed for the amount of time necessary, assist him or her to stand and step out of the tub. Provide a towel and assist the client to pat dry. Then assist the client with toilet articles, dressing, and returning to bed.
- Clean and disinfect the tub (or shower) if indicated.

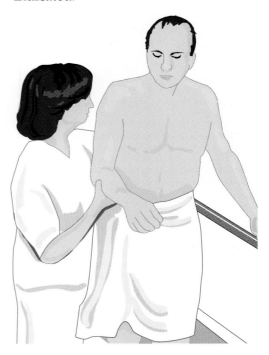

Follow the completion guidelines on pages 124-125 as indicated by the Completion Symbol. Pay special attention to the guidelines on *Personal Care* on page 187.

Shampooing Hair

Shampooing hair is necessary for good grooming. Time, frequency, and method of shampooing will differ by client. Some clients provide self-care. Others require assistance during a tub bath or shower. You can also shampoo the hair of clients in bed using a special trough to catch the water (shown below). After shampooing, you will style the client's hair as he or she likes it.

PROCEDURE

1. PREPARATION

- Follow the preparation guidelines on pages 114-115 as indicated by the Preparation Symbol. Pay special attention to the guidelines on *Personal Care* on page 187.

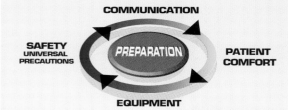

- Fill the pitcher with 110 degree water and place it with your equipment on a convenient surface. Check water temperature with a bath thermometer.
- Cover the client with the bath blanket and fold back the top linens to the foot of the bed. Provide privacy.

EQUIPMENT

- bath towels
- washcloth
- shampoo
- (hair conditioner if requested)
- bath thermometer
- water pitcher
- shampoo trough
- basin
- bath blanket
- waterproof pad
- brush and comb
- hair dryer

2. POSITION CLIENT

- With the client supine, remove pillow and move the client's head and shoulders to the side of the bed near you.
- Cover the mattress under the client's head and shoulders with the waterproof pad.
- Place the shampoo trough under the client's head and position the basin on a chair next to the bed so that runoff water will flow from the trough into the basin.

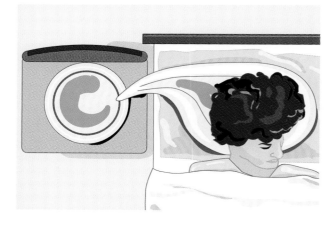

➡ *If you use a pillow to support the client's neck, cover it with a towel.*

➡ *Make sure the client is not on the edge of the bed.*

POINTERS

BRUSHING HAIR

When you brush a client's hair:

- Raise the client to a sitting position.
- Place a towel over the pillow (or over the shoulders if using a chair).
- Remove any things that could get in the way: glasses, hairpins, clips, etc.
- Gently brush the hair in sections, removing tangles.
- Style as asked.
- Carefully remove tangles. Don't pull or tug.

3. SHAMPOO

- Brush the client's hair free of tangles. Fold a face towel for the client to place over his or her eyes.
- Pour water over the hair to wet it thoroughly. Rub a small amount of shampoo into a lather from the forehead back. Massage the scalp as you lather.
- Rinse and repeat if necessary.

4. DRY AND COMPLETE

- Turban-wrap the client's head in towel. Dry his or her face with the washcloth. Remove the trough.
- Remove the wet towel and rub the hair dry with a dry towel. Comb the hair to remove tangles and dry with hair dryer. Style as requested.

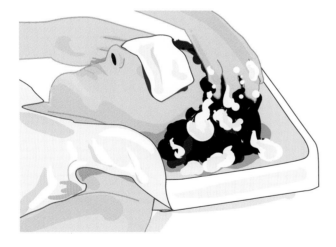

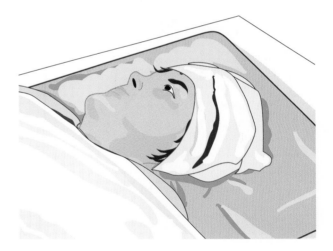

➡ *Warm the shampoo in your palms before applying it.*

➡ *Apply a hair conditioner if requested by the client. Follow the directions for the specific conditioner.*

Follow the completion guidelines on pages 124-125 as indicated by the Completion Symbol. Pay special attention to the guidelines on *Personal Care* on page 187.

Shaving Facial Hair

In shaving a male client's face, you will follow *Universal Precautions* because there is the possibility of cutting the skin. Collect the following equipment on a convenient surface: bath towel, face cloth, wash basin with 110 degree water, bath thermometer, **disposable gloves,** safety razor, mirror, shaving cream, and after shave. Check the water temperature with the bath thermometer.

PROCEDURE

1. POSITION CLIENT

- Follow the preparation guidelines (pages 114-115) and for *Personal Care* (page 187).
- Raise the client to a sitting position (if permitted) and place a bath towel over the client's chest and lower neck.
- Wash the bearded area of the face and neck with a face cloth to soften the beard. Rub shaving cream over the area. Rinse your hands.

2. SHAVE

- **Put on gloves.** Position the client's face with one hand. With the other hand, shave the beard in smooth downward strokes on the face and upward stokes on the neck and under the chin.
- Wipe clean.

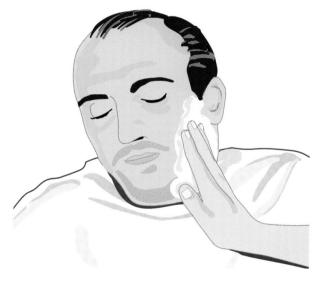

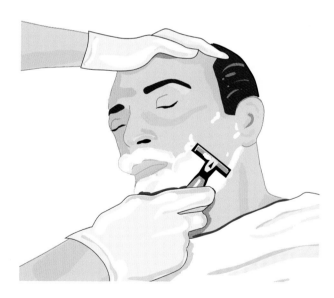

➤ *If there are any cuts or sores on the client's face, put on gloves before applying shaving cream.*

➤ *If using an electric razor, apply shaving lotion if the client requests it.*

➤ *If you cut the skin with the razor, apply direct pressure to the cut with your finger until the bleeding stops.*

➤ *Apply after-shave if requested.*

POINTERS

Nail Care

Some clients may need you to perform their nail care. **Generally, this means soaking, cleaning, and shaping—but not trimming.** Misshaped nails, diabetes, poor circulation, etc. can make trimming nails difficult or dangerous. It is usually performed by a nurse or physician. If you are allowed to trim nails and ordered to do so, use caution and follow your supervisor's instructions. When routine nail care is ordered, you will need a bath towel, wash basin, orange stick, and emery board or nail file. If you are to trim nails, you will also need disposable gloves.

1. SOAK AND CLEAN

- Follow the preparation guidelines (pages 114-115) and for *Personal Care* (page 187).

- Place a basin filled with 110 degree water on a convenient surface and position it so that the client can soak his or her fingers or feet (A.).

- Soak for ten minutes. Then pat the hands (or feet) dry. With the file or stick, carefully clean under the nails (B.).

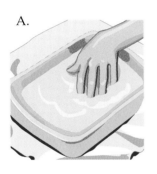

A.

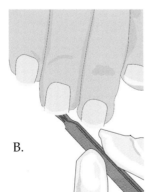

B.

2. SHAPE

- With the file or stick, gently push back the cuticle (A.).

- If ordered to trim nails, clip nails straight across with a clipper, being careful not to cut too close to the finger (B.).

- File and shape the nails with an emery board or file (C.). Follow completion guidelines on pages 124-125.

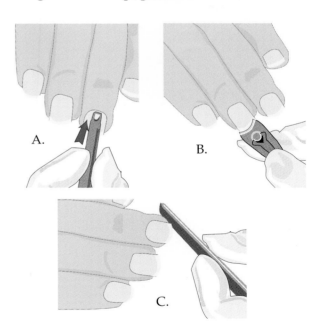

A.

B.

C.

➡ *Soaking nails in warm water first softens them and makes shaping easier.*

➡ *It is especially important to observe the condition of the toes and feet and to report any problems to your supervisor.*

Back Massage

Massaging the skin relaxes the client and stimulates circulation, which helps to prevent the development of decubitus ulcers. Your fingernails must be clipped short so you will not scratch the skin. **You will only give a back massage when it is ordered by your supervisor.** You will generally massage for 3-5 minutes.

PROCEDURE

1. PREPARATION

- Follow the preparation guidelines on pages 114-115 as indicated by the Preparation Symbol. Pay special attention to the guidelines on *Personal Care* on page 187.

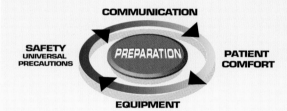

- Place the lotion in a basin of warm water.
- Assist the client to the prone or side-lying position and expose the client's back to the buttocks.
- Check skin for red areas.

EQUIPMENT

- skin lotion
- bath towel
- wash basin

2. LONG STROKE

- With your hands flat, gently rub lotion on client's back. Use a long stroke upward along the spine from the buttocks to the shoulders, turning out at the shoulders to the upper arm and stroking back toward the base of the spine.
- Repeat for at least a minute.

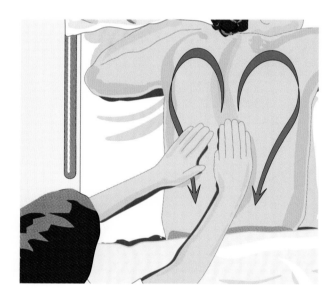

➡ *Don't rub any reddened areas.*
➡ *Use a gentle pressure and try to maintain a rhythm as you rub.*

POINTERS

3. SMALL CIRCLES

- Change the downstroke to a series of circles down the ribs to the lower back. Repeat for a minute.

4. KNEAD

- Knead the skin from the buttocks to the shoulders by gently gripping the skin with your fingertips while keeping an open hand. Repeat several times. Finish by using long strokes up and down for about a minute.

- Pat the client's back with a towel. Help the client dress and return the client to a comfortable position.

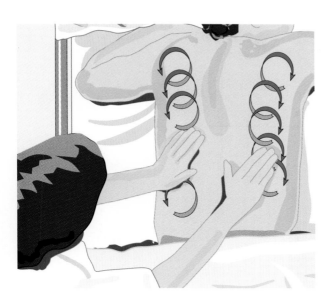

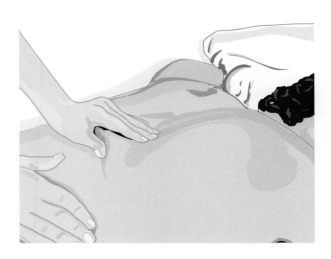

➡ *Observe the skin carefully and report any unusual conditions.*

➡ *Use a gentle pressure and try to maintain a rhythm as you rub.*

Follow the completion guidelines on pages 124-125 as indicated by the Completion Symbol. Pay special attention to the guidelines on *Personal Care* on page 187.

Dressing and Undressing Clients

When assisting in dressing and undressing clients, you must provide privacy, encourage self-care, and allow clients to select their clothes whenever appropriate. Remember that clothing is a form of self-expression. Respect the client's preferences and show a positive attitude about them. Use this opportunity to talk with the client.

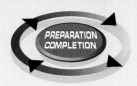

Follow these guidelines (as well as regular preparation and completion guidelines) when assisting clients to dress and undress:

✔ Provide privacy.

✔ Encourage self-care.

✔ Accommodate client preferences regarding dressing and clothes as much as possible.

✔ Make sure clothing is clean and neat.

✔ Dress and undress the upper body first.

✔ Dress a client's weak side first.

✔ Provide help as it is needed.

✔ Observe the client for signs of dizziness, unsteadiness, or other problems.

✔ Observe the client's skin condition.

✔ Make sure footwear is put on **before** the client gets out of bed and that it fits comfortably.

✔ Follow your supervisor's instructions regarding soiled clothing. Make sure that clothing that will be worn again is properly stored (in closets, on hangers, in dressers, etc.).

Show a positive attitude about the client's appearance and compliment it when appropriate.

UNDRESSING WITH AN IV

● Assist the client to a sitting position. Take shirts or blouses off the arm **opposite the IV.** Provide a bath blanket for the client to hold over his or her chest.

● Roll the garment to the IV side, down the arm, and over the hand.

● Remove the IV from the IV pole and slip it through the sleeve of the client's garment. Hang the IV back on the IV pole.

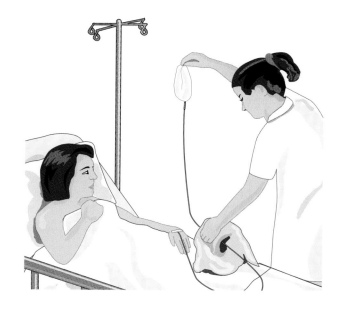

➡ *Keep the IV above the level of the client's arm so you won't affect the flow of IV fluid.*

➡ *Reverse these steps to put on a garment.*

POINTERS

208

PUTTING ON PANTS

- Assist the client to sit on the edge of the bed.
- Put on underwear, socks or stockings, and pants. Pull the socks or stockings completely up and the underwear and pants as high as the thighs.
- Put on shoes and assist the client to stand. Help the client pull underwear and pants up the rest of the way. Fasten pants.

REMOVING PANTS

- Remove shoes or slippers and assist clients to the supine position. Unfasten pants.
- Ask clients to raise their hips off the bed by pushing off with their feet. Slide pants off the hips. The hips can then be lowered to the bed.
- Remove pants the rest of the way. Handle soiled clothes as directed. Hang clean clothes up.

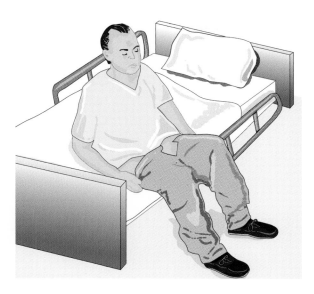

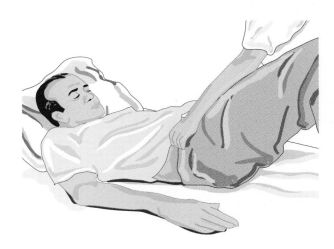

➡ *Be sure to use good body mechanics when helping the client to stand.*

➡ *If you have to put pants on a supine client, ask the client to raise his or her hips off the bed while you slip the pants over the hips.*

➡ *Pajama bottoms are removed the same way.*

➡ *If a client can't raise his or her hips off the bed, remove pants one side at a time by having the client turn in the side-lying position.*

Personal Care

1.
Describe how a bath or shower makes you feel physically. Does it affect your attitude as well? If so, how? What about a clean change of clothing?

2.
Beginning with the start of the day, list as many of your personal care habits as you can: how and when you like to bathe, shampoo, brush your teeth, change clothes, etc. Are there any habits that it would bother you to change? Which ones? Why?

3.
In what ways do you notice the personal hygiene and grooming of others? How does this influence your opinion of them?

4.
If you needed someone to perform your personal care, what guidelines would you give them? How would you like them to treat you?

REVIEW

**Key Terms – Test your understanding of each of these first.
Then use each one once to fill in the incomplete statements below.**

universal precautions

flossing

oral care

dentures

bed bath

105-110 degrees

perineal care

tub bath or shower

shampooing

massaging

1. Clients who must stay in bed are given a _____, in which the client's entire body is washed a part at a time.

2. After _____, you will brush the client's hair as they like it.

3. _____ is provided every two hours to unconscious clients to keep them from aspirating saliva.

4. You must practice _____ when providing oral hygiene or shaving a client because of the possibility of coming in contact with the client's blood.

5. When assisting a client taking a _____ you must be alert to safety hazards such as slippery surfaces, overly hot water, or temporary dizziness.

6. _____the skin relaxes the client and stimulates circulation, which helps to prevent the development of decubitus ulcers.

7. _____ are false teeth that are form-fitted to the gums and must be cleaned as often as natural teeth.

8. _____ is a safe temperature range for bathing water.

9. _____ teeth removes tartar and food particles from surfaces difficult to clean with a toothbrush.

10. _____ involves cleaning the genitals, anus, and the area between (the *perineum*).

Elimination

Assisting clients to eliminate will be one of your basic responsibilities.

The act of eliminating solid waste (*feces or stool*) is called *defecation* or having a *bowel movement*. The act of eliminating liquid waste (*urine*) is called *voiding*. For most people, these are regular and automatic activities. However, many clients are unable to eliminate comfortably and safely without assistance and will need your help.

Many people have difficulties with elimination.

Age, disease, and diet can affect the body's ability to eliminate waste normally. Some clients may experience pain or discomfort as a symptom of a disorder. *Constipation* is a condition where bowel movements are difficult to have and may be hard and painful. *Incontinence* is an inability to control the release of urine and sometimes feces.

Assisting elimination requires prompt action and special sensitivity.

Clients may find the need for assistance irritating, embarrassing, or depressing. In addition, as the urge to defecate or void can happen quickly (often the result of eating, drinking, or taking medication), delays in assistance can cause discomfort, incontinence, and further embarrassment. It can also lead to falls when clients who need assistance try to use the bathroom without any help.

You will be responsible for monitoring elimination and recognizing problems or abnormal results.

You will often be required to measure output and report observations. Normal urine is clear pale yellow with a faint smell. Normal feces is brown and should be soft but formed. Urine or feces that is discolored or has an overpowering odor or unusual appearance may be abnormal and must be reported.

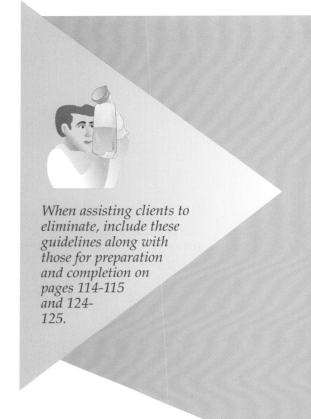

When assisting clients to eliminate, include these guidelines along with those for preparation and completion on pages 114-115 and 124-125.

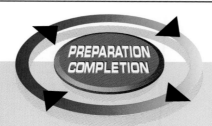

PREPARATION
COMPLETION

Communication

✔ Learn what words the client uses to describe elimination and if they are appropriate use them.

Client Comfort

✔ Respond to requests for assistance promptly. The urge to eliminate often requires quick action.

✔ Offer frequently to assist clients to eliminate so they are not forced to ask for your help.

✔ **Be alert to incontinence.** Change linens and wash affected areas of clients.

✔ Make sure the client has complete privacy. Close doors, pull curtains closed, cover client with bath towel, etc.

Equipment

✔ Always keep an extra set of disposable gloves in case you need them.

✔ Always clean and disinfect urinals, bedpans, commodes, and any other equipment when finished.

✔ Make sure toilet paper is conveniently placed for clients performing self-care.

Safety

✔ **Wear gloves and follow Universal Precautions** any time you might come in contact with blood or body fluids (feces, urine, semen, vaginal secretions, etc.).

✔ Use aseptic techniques with all contaminated equipment and materials.

✔ Make sure floors are dry when assisting clients to use a bedside commode or the bathroom.

✔ Use good body mechanics when lifting or supporting clients.

Assisting with a Bedpan

Clients confined to bed will use a bedpan when having a bowel movement. Female clients will also use a bedpan to void. You will place a bedpan underneath the client, raise the client to a sitting position, and provide privacy. **Practice Universal Precautions and be alert to incontinence when assisting client elimination.** You will often be required to measure client output and report on its appearance.

PROCEDURE

1. PREPARATION

- Follow the preparation guidelines on pages 114-115 as indicated by the Preparation Symbol. Pay special attention to the guidelines on *Elimination* on page 213.

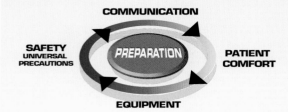

- If using a hospital bed, put the bed in the horizontal position at a comfortable height for you to work.
- If using side rails, remove or lower them on the side you will stand. The rail on the far side should be raised for safety.

EQUIPMENT

- standard bedpan or fracture pan (see above right)
- bedpan cover or towel
- toilet paper
- disposable gloves
- waterproof pad
- paper towels
- wash cloth
- face towel
- wash basin
- soap

2a. POSITION PAN

- Pull back the top linens.
- Ask the client to raise his or her hips off the bed by pushing off the mattress with the feet.
- Slide the waterproof pad and pan under the client's buttocks. Position the pan so all waste will be eliminated into it.

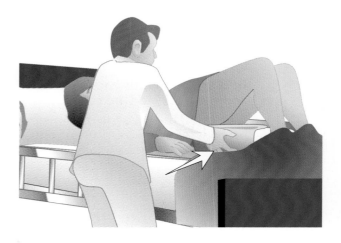

➡ *The buttocks sit on the flat end of the bedpan.*

➡ *Be alert to incontinence. Put on disposable gloves immediately if the client has been incontinent.*

POINTERS

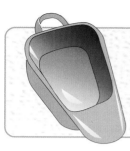

FRACTURE PANS

Sometimes you will need to use a *fracture pan* for clients who find moving in bed difficult. The fracture pan is smaller than a standard bedpan and has one very shallow end. The shallow end is slid gently under the buttocks so that the client moves as little as possible.

2b. ROLLING CLIENT

- If the client cannot raise his or her hips so you can slide the bedpan underneath them, turn the client to a side-lying position facing away from you.
- Place the bedpan flat against the buttocks.
- Assist the client to roll gently back onto the pan. Make sure you hold the pan in place as the client rolls onto it.

3. POSITION CLIENT

- With the client on the bedpan, raise him or her to a sitting position—use pillows for support if necessary. Replace top linens. Raise side rail if one is used.
- Place toilet paper within easy reach. Provide privacy and leave to wash hands.
- Return in five minutes to check, or sooner if called.

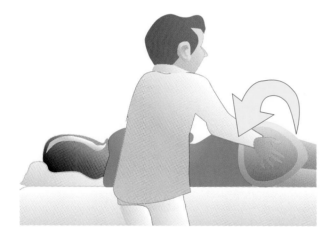

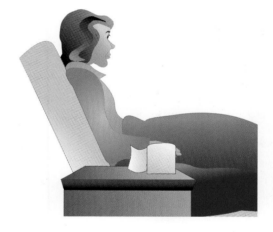

➡ *Sitting helps to empty the bladder and bowels.*

➡ *Running water in the client's sink can often help stimulate urination.*

➡ *Make sure the pan is positioned so that all waste will be eliminated directly into the pan.*

Assisting with a Bedpan (Cont'd)

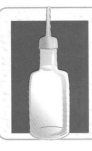

ENEMAS

An enema creates an urge to defecate by the injection of fluid into the rectum. A **cleansing enema** injects a cleansing solution into the rectum which the client eliminates along with feces a short time later. **Commercial enemas** come in ready-to-use squeezeable containers (shown at left). Since enemas can have harmful effects, however, **home care aides are often not allowed to administer them. Learn and follow your agency's policy on enemas.**

PROCEDURE

4. REMOVE PAN

- **Wash hands and put on disposable gloves.**
- Remove the bedpan by reversing the procedure: pull back top linens and assist the client off the bedpan the same way he or she got on it.

5. CLEAN CLIENT

- Cover the bedpan and place on a nearby surface, being careful not to spill the contents.
- If necessary, assist the client to wipe. **Wiping should be performed in the same manner as perineal care (front to back).** See the procedure on pages 198-199.
- Provide perineal care if needed. Remove waterproof pad.

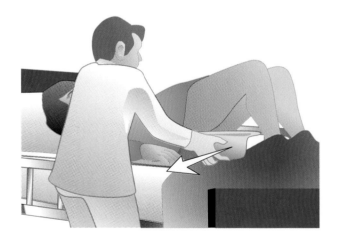

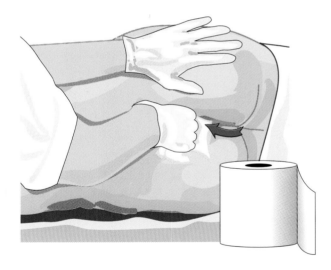

➡ *If the client is to roll off the bedpan, secure the bedpan with one hand as you assist the client to turn with the other.*

➡ *Prepare enough paper before beginning so you will not contaminate roll with soiled gloves.*

➡ *Handle the bedpan with extreme care. Wipe up any spills and disinfect contaminated areas immediately.*

POINTERS

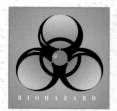

BIOHAZARD

Urine or stool are potentially contagious and require the practice of Universal Precautions and aseptic technique. You must take special care to protect your clients, co-workers, and yourself, following the guidelines on Infection Control on pages 88-89 and on Gloves and Contaminated Material on pages 120-123.

6. DISPOSE AND DISINFECT

- Dispose of waste according to agency guidelines.
- Observe output and measure if indicated.
- Clean and disinfect the bedpan and return to bedside stand with clean cover. Remove gloves.

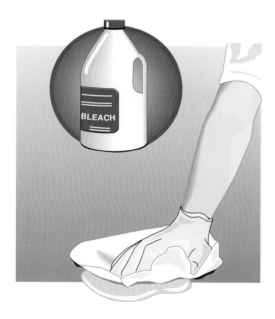

➡ *Always observe color, appearance, and odor of client urine and stool. Report abnormalities to your supervisor. Do not dispose of abnormal urine and stool until after reporting.*

7. COMPLETION

- Assist the client to wash his or her hands. Use handi-wipes or a clean washcloth, soap, and warm (110 degree) water.
- Position client comfortably. Remove soiled linens. Wash your hands. If making the bed, follow the procedure for *Making an Occupied Bed* on pages 152-155.

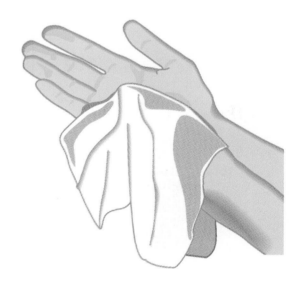

Follow the completion guidelines on pages 124-125 as indicated by the Completion Symbol. Pay special attention to the guidelines on *Elimination* on page 213.

Using a Bedside Commode

Clients who can stand but not walk to a bathroom may eliminate into a portable bedside commode with a removable pan. You assist the client to and from the bedside commode as you would to a wheelchair. **Follow the preparation and completion steps for** *Assisting with a Bedpan* **(pages 214-217), using a commode instead of a bedpan and waterproof pad. Then follow the steps below.**

See pages 214-217

PROCEDURE

1. POSITION CLIENT

- Check to make sure the pan is securely in place before seating the client on the commode.

- Assist the client to sit and place a bath blanket over his or her lap for privacy. Place toilet paper within easy reach of the client. Provide privacy.

- Wash your hands. Return in five minutes to check, or sooner if called.

2. COMPLETION AND DISPOSAL

- When the client is finished, wash your hands and put on disposable gloves. Assist the client to clean the perineal area if needed and return him or her to bed.

- Remove the pan and cover. Empty, clean, and disinfect according to agency guidelines. Replace in the commode. Remove gloves and wash hands.

- Assist the client to wash his or her hands.

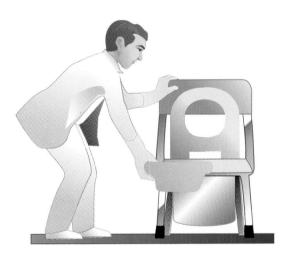

➡ *See pages 176-177 for assisting the client to a chair.*
➡ *Remember to lock the wheels of the commode.*

➡ *Handle the bedpan with extreme care. Wipe up any spills and disinfect contaminated areas immediately (commode seat, bedpan, etc.).*

POINTERS

218

Using a Urinal

A urinal is used by male clients who cannot walk to a bathroom. The client urinates into the urinal while in bed or standing next to it. **Follow the preparation and completion steps for** *Assisting with a Bedpan* **(pages 214-217), using a urinal instead of a bedpan and waterproof pad. Then follow the steps below.**

1. POSITION THE CLIENT

- Raise the client in bed to a sitting position and pull back the top linens.

- The client should place the urinal between his legs and insert his penis into the opening to urinate. **If he needs your assistance to do this, put on gloves first.**

- Replace top linens and provide privacy. Wash your hands before leaving.

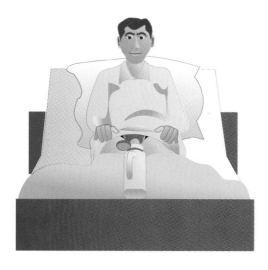

➡ *Assisting the client to sit on the side of the bed will make it easier to empty the bladder. If he still has difficulty, assist the client to stand. However, make sure the client is not dizzy. Stay with him until he finishes.*

2. COMPLETION AND DISPOSAL

- When the client is finished, he may place the cover on the urinal and place it on a convenient surface.

- Return in five minutes to check, or sooner if called. Wash your hands and put on disposable gloves. Help the client wash his hands. Empty, clean, and disinfect the urinal and any contaminated surfaces.

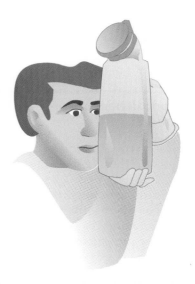

➡ *Observe color, appearance, and odor of client's urine. Report abnormal urine to your supervisor.*

➡ *The urinal should be stored within the client's reach so it can be used by the client at his convenience.*

Urinary Catheters

> An *indwelling urinary catheter* is a tube inserted into the bladder that will drain urine out of it.

Also called a *retention* or *Foley* catheter, it is inserted through the urethra and held in place inside the bladder by the inflation of a small balloon at its tip. Urine automatically flows through the tube to a drainage bag that is placed below the level of the bladder.

> The indwelling catheter and drainage bag are a closed system that can be contaminated through handling.

Because bacteria grow easily in urine, there is a strong risk of infection if the catheter and drainage bag are mishandled. The catheter is generally taped to the client's inner thigh to secure it. Never pull on it and always handle it with great care any time the client is moved in or out of bed.

> Only nurses and physicians may insert an indwelling catheter.

The home care aide is responsible for checking the catheter, keeping it and the client clean, and emptying the drainage bag. **Because you will be exposed to body fluids, you must use Universal Precautions and wear disposable gloves.** Catheter care (cleaning the client and the catheter) is provided daily during pericare or whenever necessary. The drainage bag is emptied at least once every eight hours.

CATHETER POSITIONING

- The catheter is taped to the inside of the thigh to secure it.
- **Never hang extra tubing in a loop between the client and the bag.** Extra tubing should be coiled flat on the bed and secured with a tube clip.
- The drainage bag must be lower than the bladder. It may be hung on a bed frame, wheelchair frame, or taped to the client's leg. **Never attach the drainage bag to side rails.**

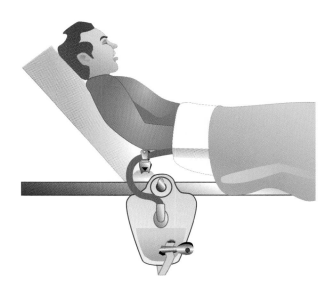

➥ *Urine must flow freely in the catheter. Tubing should never be bent or kinked.*

➥ *Never let the catheter or the drainage bag touch the floor.*

POINTERS

CLEANING CLIENT

- **Prepare as in Step 1 of *Perineal Care* on page 198. Put on gloves.**
- Check for any leakage, secretions, or irritation. Spread the labia of females. Pull back the foreskin of uncircumcised males.
- Gently clean the area around the *meatus* (the urethral opening) using an applicator or soap, water and a clean washcloth. Rinse and pat dry.

CLEANING CATHETER

- With a sterile wipe (or clean washcloth and soap and water), clean four inches of the catheter by gently wiping away from where it enters the meatus.
- Continue with pericare or finish by removing the waterproof pad and following the completion guidelines on pages 124-125 and the *Elimination* guidelines on page 213.

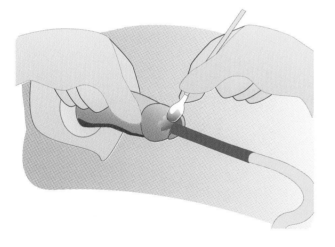

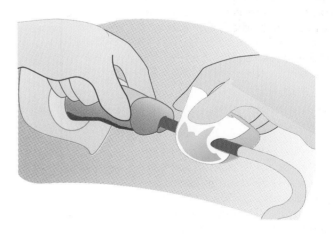

➡ *A cleaning kit with applicators is often used.*

➡ *A gentle touch is necessary to prevent irritation.*

➡ ***Never pull on catheter tubing.***

➡ ***Remember to use Universal Precautions and aseptic practices.***

Applying a Condom Catheter

An external catheter called a condom catheter is sometimes used on incontinent male clients to contain urine leakage. It fits over the tip of the penis. It is often used with a small drainage bag that attaches to the leg (*leg bag*) and allows the client to get out of bed. Home care aides may apply a condom catheter when ordered by a nurse or physician. It is replaced daily.

APPLICATION

- Follow manufacturer's instructions, preparation guidelines on pages 114-115, and the *Elimination* guidelines on page 213. **Put on gloves.**

- With the client supine, uncover the penis and apply a skin barrier to the shaft. Unroll the condom end of the catheter smoothly over the penis and skin barrier. Gently press the catheter against the skin barrier.

- Secure the drainage bag to the leg or bed frame. Connect the condom end to the tubing and the drainage bag.

CLEANING

- Prepare as in Step 1 of *Perineal Care* on page 198.

- Gently unroll the condom end and the skin barrier off the penis. Detach from tubing and dispose.

- Provide pericare as in step 2.b on page 199. Pay close attention to the condition of the skin. Follow completion guidelines on pages 124-125 and the *Elimination* guidelines on page 213.

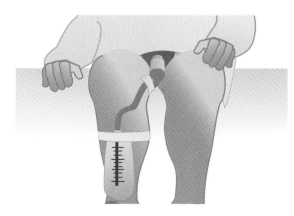

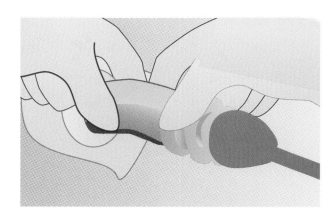

➥ *Follow the manufacturer's directions carefully for applying the skin barrier and condom. Report any broken or irritated skin to your supervisor immediately.*

➥ *Make sure there are no kinks in the tubing so urine will flow freely.*

➥ *Check leg bags every two hours.*

➥ *Make sure to wash off any skin barrier residue. Observe the condition of the skin. Report any broken or irritated skin to your supervisor immediately.*

Emptying a Drainage Bag

Standard drainage bags are emptied at least once every eight hours. Leg bags are much smaller and must be checked every two hours. You will carefully empty the drainage bag into a graduate or measuring cup. **Use *Universal Precautions* and aseptic technique because of the risk of infection.** Then observe, measure, record and dispose of the output.

1. POSITION SPOUT

- Follow preparation guidelines on pages 114-115 and the *Elimination* guidelines on page 213.
- Put on gloves. Place the graduate on the floor directly below the drainage bag.
- Detach the spout from its holder and point it into the center of the graduate.

2. DRAIN AND REPLACE

- Unclamp the spout and empty the drainage bag into the graduate.
- When the bag is empty, clamp the spout and clean the tip with an antiseptic wipe. Replace in holder.
- Observe, measure, record and dispose of the output. Clean the graduate and return it to its place.

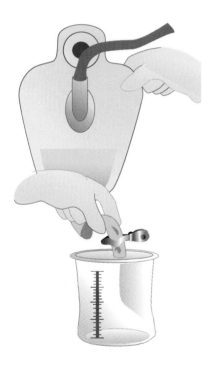

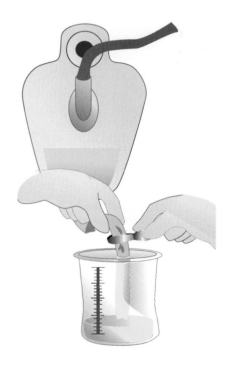

➡ *Be careful not to contaminate the spout by touching the sides of the graduate with it.*

Follow completion guidelines on pages 124-125 and the *Elimination* guidelines on page 213.

Ostomy Care

An *ostomy* is a surgically created opening (called a *stoma*) through the abdomen to the digestive tract. It can be permanent or temporary. Liquid and solid waste leave the digestive tract through the stoma. They are collected in a disposable pouch called an *appliance* that is worn on the abdomen. Initial ostomy care is performed by nurses but home care aides and clients may be directed to provide care if the ostomy is permanent. **Use Universal Precautions when providing ostomy care.**

PROCEDURE

1. PREPARATION

- Follow the preparation guidelines on pages 114-115 as indicated by the Preparation Symbol. Pay special attention to the guidelines on *Elimination* on page 213.

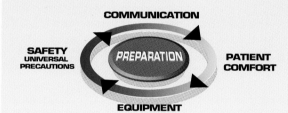

- There are many types of ostomies and ostomy equipment. If you are directed to perform ostomy care, follow manufacturer's directions and the instructions of a supervising nurse or physician.

EQUIPMENT

- disposable gloves
- ostomy appliance
- ostomy belt
- wafer and adhesive skin barrier
- bed protector pads
- gauze wipes and wash cloth
- soap or skin cleanser
- hypoallergenic tape
- bedpan with cover
- toilet tissue
- bath blanket
- wash basin
- bath thermometer
- waste bag

2. REMOVE APPLIANCE

- Cover the client with a bath blanket. Then lift the blanket to uncover the appliance. Place a bed protector under the hips.
- **Put on gloves.** Gently detach the appliance from the belt. Remove the belt.
- Carefully lift the appliance off the wafer. Place the appliance in the bedpan. Gently peel the wafer and adhesive barrier away from the skin.

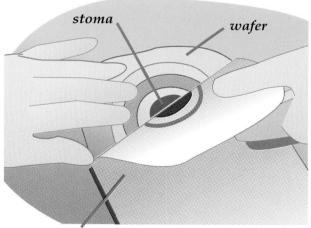

➥ *Appliances should be emptied when one-third full or according to agency policy.*

➥ *Some appliances are designed to be reused (following manufacturer's directions) after careful cleaning with an antiseptic solution.*

POINTERS

NOTES ON OSTOMIES

- Some appliances can be drained into a toilet or bedpan while still worn by unclamping the appliance opening. When drained, the opening is wiped with an antiseptic wipe and clamped.

- Waste is less liquid and closer to normal the closer the stoma is to the lower end of the large intestine.

- A *colostomy* creates an opening to the colon. An *iliostomy* creates an opening to the small intestine.

3. CLEAN AROUND STOMA

- Wipe away any waste around the stoma with a gauze pad or tissue.

- Wet a clean washcloth in 105-110 degree water and place it over the stoma and surrounding area. Allow enough time to loosen any remaining adhesive.

- When the adhesive is loosened, remove the washcloth and gently wash the skin around the stoma, working from the cleanest to the dirtiest area. Use a gauze wipe and an oil-free soap.

4. ATTACH APPLIANCE

- Once the skin is completely clean and dry, apply the skin barrier and adhesive to the skin around the stoma according to the manufacturer's instructions. The wafer should seal to the skin.

- Attach the appliance. Use hypoallergenic tape to secure if necessary.

- Put a clean belt on the client. Attach appliance to belt.

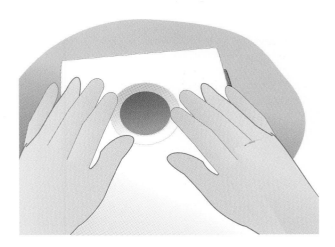

➥ *Waste matter contains acids and enzymes that irritate the skin as well as potentially infectious pathogens. Report any signs of skin irritation to your supervisor immediately.*

➥ *Oily or creamy soaps can prevent the skin barrier from sticking to the skin.*

Follow the completion guidelines on pages 124-125 as indicated by the Completion Symbol. Pay special attention to the guidelines on *Elimination* on page 213.

COMPLETION

Elimination

1.
How would you feel about discussing your own elimination habits with others?

2.
How would you feel about other people observing and testing your feces and urine?

3.
How would you feel about needing someone's assistance to eliminate?

4.
How do you think you would feel if you suffered from incontinence?

REVIEW

**Key Terms – Test your understanding of each of these first.
Then use each one once to fill in the incomplete statements below.**

feces

urine

urge to eliminate

constipation

incontinence

discoloration

bedpan

bedside commode

urinal

catheter

stoma

appliance

enema

1. Liquid and solid waste leave the digestive tract of clients with ostomies through a _____ and are collected in an _____ worn around the waist.

2. Clients confined to bed will use a _____ to void or have a bowel movement.

3. An indwelling urinary _____ is a tube inserted into the bladder through which urine drains to a drainage bag.

4. _____ is a condition where bowel movements are difficult to have and may be hard and painful.

5. _____ is solid waste from the intestines. _____ is liquid waste from the urinary system.

6. _____, strong odor, or unusual appearance of urine and feces are abnormalities that must be reported.

7. An _____ is the artificial creation of an urge to defecate by the injection of fluid into the rectum.

8. The _____ can happen quickly and requires prompt action.

9. Clients capable of standing but not walking to a bathroom may eliminate into a portable _____ with a removable pan.

10. _____ is an inability to control the release of urine and sometimes feces.

11. Male clients who cannot walk to the bathroom may void in a _____.

Specimen Collection

A client's care may require analysis of blood, body fluid, and waste samples.

Home care aides often collect samples (called *specimens*) of their clients' urine, feces, and *sputum* (mucous from the lungs and bronchial tubes). They may also perform simple urine tests. They are generally **not** allowed to collect blood specimens.

Collecting specimens accurately is essential.

A specimen improperly collected or mishandled can result in a wrong diagnosis and incorrect treatment of a client. Specimens must be clearly labeled and properly collected. If a mistake is made in collection, the specimen must be thrown away and a new specimen taken.

Specimens are potentially infectious.

Always use Universal Precautions and aseptic technique when collecting and handling specimens (see pages 88-89 and 116-123) so you do not infect yourself or others.

Prompt and careful handling is required.

Careless handling can contaminate the specimen and spread infection. Some specimens may require refrigeration or other special handling. Be sure to know and follow your agency's policy regarding storing and forwarding specimens.

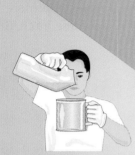

When collecting specimens, include these guidelines along with those for preparation and completion on pages 114-115 and assisting elimination on pages 212-213.

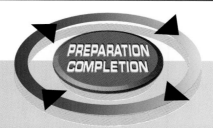

Communication

✔ Make sure the client understands what is expected and why. If the client does not understand, you may get a contaminated or incorrect sample and have to start over.

✔ Learn to recognize normal and abnormal elimination for each client.

✔ Learn your agency's labeling and reporting policy. Clearly identify and record all the information required.

✔ Double-check all information to guarantee accuracy. **If there is any doubt in your mind, throw away the specimen,** begin over, and report it to your supervisor.

Client Comfort

✔ Be especially sensitive to the client's feelings when discussing or collecting specimens.

✔ Observe client for physical discomfort during elimination and report instances to your supervisor.

✔ Be alert to the need for fresh linens, skin care, pericare, etc.

Equipment

✔ Learn your agency's guidelines on using specimen collection equipment. Know how everything is used, where to get it or take it, what is disposable and reusable, etc.

Safety

✔ **Always wear disposable gloves and use Universal Precautions and aseptic technique.**

✔ Be careful not to touch the inside surfaces of specimen containers and lids as this will contaminate the specimen.

✔ Keep the outside surfaces of specimen containers from being contaminated by the specimens.

✔ Handle and process specimens promptly and according to agency policy.

✔ Always dispose of disposable items and process reusable items according to your agency's policy.

Routine Urine Specimen

Different types of urine specimens are collected. Many clients will collect their own specimens. You may perform simple tests on urine specimens or have to forward them for analysis. Some specimens require clients to start and stop voiding at will. All specimens must be free of feces, toilet paper, and other material. Whatever type of specimen you are collecting, you must carefully explain the procedure to the client and ask for his or her cooperation. **Use Universal Precautions.**

PROCEDURE

1. PREPARATION

- Follow the preparation guidelines on pages 114-115 as indicated by the Preparation Symbol. Pay special attention to the guidelines on *Elimination* on page 213 and on *Specimen Collection* on page 229.

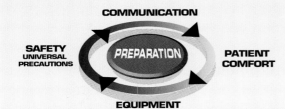

- Fill out the specimen label with the client's name and the time and date. Place the label on the container.

EQUIPMENT

- Bedpan and cover, urinal, specimen pan
- Specimen container with lid
- Specimen label
- Disposable gloves
- Plastic bag
- Toilet tissue

➡ *If testing for sugar or acetone in urine, you will use tablets or strips that react with the urine to produce a color. The color indicates the reading. Follow the manufacturer's instructions for the test you are using.*

2. COLLECT URINE

- **Put on gloves.** If necessary, assist the client to void into a bedpan, urinal, or specimen pan following the elimination procedures on pages 214-219. (A specimen pan is placed over the toilet opening under the toilet seat to catch elimination.)

- Ask clients not to defecate into the bedpan or specimen pan or place toilet tissue into it. Provide a plastic bag for toilet tissue.

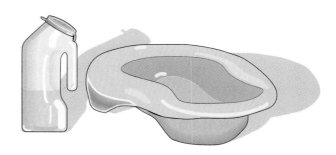

➡ *Wear disposable gloves and use aseptic technique and Universal Precautions.*

POINTERS

FRESH-FRACTIONAL

Two urine specimens (in two containers) are taken 30 minutes apart, the second being the *fresh-fractional* urine. The first specimen is analyzed, but the second specimen is the important one. If producing fresh urine in 30 minutes is impossible, the results of the first specimen may have to be used but noted as *"not fresh-fractional."* You will use a fresh-fractional specimen for a sugar or acetone test.

3. TRANSFER URINE

- Take the urine to the client's bathroom or other approved location. Measure output if indicated.
- Pour urine into the specimen container until it is three-quarters full.
- Place lid on specimen container and close.

4. FORWARD SPECIMEN

- Dispose of remaining urine.
- Store or forward the specimen according to agency guidelines. Be sure the label on the container has the correct client information.

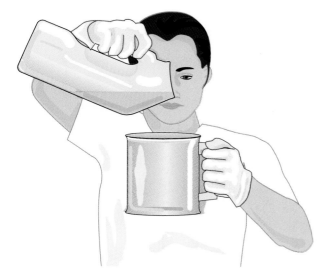

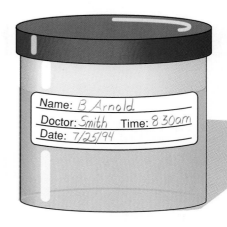

➡ *If the client is on I&O, measure the urine according to the procedure on page 143 before pouring it into the specimen container.*

➡ **As you handle the container and lid, be careful not to touch the inside surfaces as this will contaminate them.**

Follow the completion guidelines on pages 124-125 as indicated by the Completion Symbol. Pay special attention to the guidelines on *Elimination* on page 213 and on *Specimen Collection* on page 229.

Midstream Clean-Catch

Urine picks up bacteria as it travels out the urethra during voiding. A clean-catch specimen requires cleaning the perineal area and taking urine from the middle of the urine stream. The client begins voiding into a bedpan, urinal, or toilet, but stops before finishing. He or she then voids into a specimen container. To prevent contamination of the urine, the labia of females and the foreskins of uncircumcised males are held back. **Use Universal Precautions.**

PROCEDURE

1. PERICARE, THEN VOID

- **Put on gloves.** Follow step 1 of *Routine Urine Specimen* on page 230.
- Clean around the client's perineal area following steps 1, 2.a, and 2.b on pages 198-199.
- Ask the client to **hold back the foreskin or labia.** If the client cannot, you must do it. Ask the client to begin voiding but to stop before emptying the bladder.

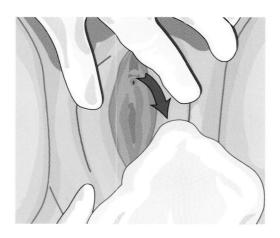

2. MIDSTREAM CLEAN-CATCH

- Ask the client to hold the specimen container so it will catch urine and to begin voiding into it. Hold the container yourself if the client can't.
- When the container is three-quarters full, ask the client to stop. Remove the container and close the lid. The client may then finish voiding.
- Follow step 4 of *Routine Urine Specimen* on page 231.

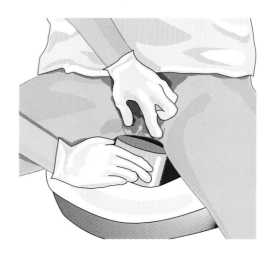

➡ *If the client cannot stop voiding, the container will have to be positioned and removed as quickly and neatly as possible.*

➡ *As you handle the container and lid, be careful not to touch the inside surfaces as this will contaminate them.*

POINTERS

➡ *You must be ready to go immediately to Step 2 in the event the client cannot stop voiding.*

➡ *Many clients can perform this procedure very well if given good instructions.*

24-Hour Specimen

Urine is collected for 24-hours, generally beginning after the client has voided at the start of the day. As urine is collected, it is poured into a large container that is sometimes refrigerated or kept on ice to prevent bacteria growth. **You will have to explain 24-hr collection carefully to your clients and their families since they will have to collect urine while you are not there.** Begin by following Step 1 of *Routine Urine Specimen* on page 230 and assemble a 24-hr container (with identification label), funnel, and ice-bucket (if indicated) in the client's bathroom or other convenient location. **Use Universal Precautions.**

1. POST NOTICES

- Create 24 hour collection notices and place in the client's room and bathroom. Label the collection container. Note start and finish times on all labels and notices.

- Have the client void to start the 24-hr period and **dispose of the urine.**

- Inform the client and his or her family that all urine for the next 24 hours will be collected.

2. 24-HOUR COLLECTION

- **Wear gloves to collect urine.** Pour urine into the collection container using a funnel. Place the container on ice or in a refrigerator, if ordered.

- At the end of 24 hours, the client should void to complete the specimen. Pour into 24-hour container, close, and forward specimen according to your agency's policy.

- Remove notices and complete procedure following *Completion* and *Specimen Collection* guidelines.

B. Arnold
24 HOUR COLLECTION
SAVE ALL URINE
7:10 A.M., 7/25 – 7:10 A.M., 7/26

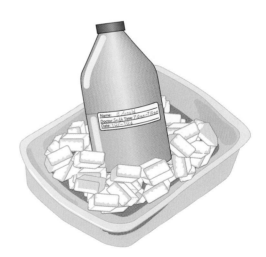

➡ *Make sure you know whether the specimen requires refrigeration. Some do.*

➡ *Ask clients not to defecate into the bedpan or specimen pan or place toilet tissue into it. Provide a plastic bag for toilet tissue.*

➡ *If using ice, replace it as it melts.*

➡ *If the client is on I&O, urine must be measured **before** pouring it into the specimen container.*

Stool Specimen

When stool specimens are collected, clients defecate into a bedpan or specimen pan **without urinating.** When a client is ready to move his or her bowels, follow the complete procedure for using a bedpan or bedside commode on pages 214-218 to produce a specimen. Explain that he or she **must not urinate into the pan** and must dispose of toilet tissue into a trash bag or toilet. **Use Universal Precautions.**

PROCEDURE

1. EQUIPMENT

- To take a stool specimen, you'll need a wooden tongue blade, disposable gloves, and a specimen container with label. Fill out the label with client information. **Put on disposable gloves.**

- You should also be prepared for the client to have a strong urge to urinate and provide a urinal.

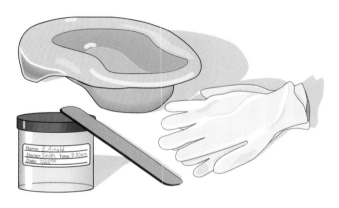

2. SCOOP SPECIMEN

- When the client is finished, scoop the amount of stool indicated (generally about 2 tablespoons) with a wooden tongue blade. Place it in the specimen container and close the lid.

- Follow completion directions of Step 4 of *Routine Urine Specimen* on page 231, disposing of the tongue blade and the remaining feces.

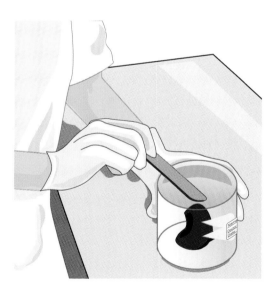

POINTERS

➡ *A specimen pan fits over the opening to the toilet: lift the toilet seat and place the pan over the opening to catch the stool.*

➡ *If you do not have a bedpan or specimen pan, ask your supervisor for advice on a substitute.*

➡ *Be sensitive to the client's feelings. They may find this procedure especially embarassing.*

➡ *Follow your supervisor's instructions on forwarding the specimen for analysis.*

Sputum Specimen

When collecting sputum specimens, the client coughs up *(expectorates)* mucous from the bronchial tubes and lungs (see pages 64-65 and 276-277). Expectorating sputum can be physically difficult and disagreeable and is generally easiest at the start of the day. It can also be noisy and embarrassing to the client and requires special sensitivity on your part. Note that sputum is thick and sometimes colored. Saliva is watery and clear. **Use Universal Precautions.**

1. PREPARE CLIENT

- To collect a sputum specimen, follow Preparation guidelines on pages 114-115 and Specimen Collection guidelines on page 229 and assemble a specimen container with label, tissues, cup of water, small basin, and disposable gloves. Fill out the label with client information. **Put on gloves.**

- Have the client rinse his or her mouth with water and spit it into the basin.

2. EXPECTORATE

- Give the client the specimen container and tissue. Ask the client to hold the tissue over the mouth and nose, inhale deeply three times, and cough up sputum. See the procedure for *Coughing and Deep-Breathing* on pages 276-277 for more information.

- Ask the client to spit the sputum into the container and continue the process until you have collected about a tablespoon. Close the lid and place container in specimen bag.

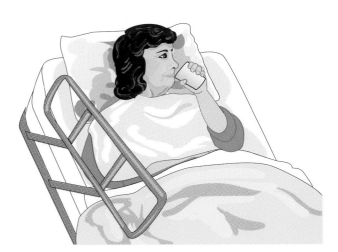

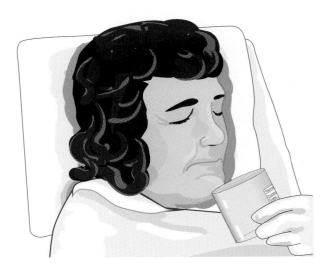

Follow the completion guidelines on pages 124-125 as indicated by the Completion Symbol. Pay special attention to the guidelines on *Specimen Collection* on page 229. Deliver or forward the specimen with requisition slip to the laboratory.

➡ *Do not use mouthwash to rinse the client's mouth as it may affect the sample.*

Specimen Collection

1.
Consider the procedure for taking a midstream clean-catch specimen and list all the ways you could:
1.) contaminate the client;
2.) contaminate yourself;
3.) contaminate others directly or indirectly.

2.
How would you feel about having your urine and stool examined and analyzed? Would it affect your ability to eliminate?

3.
If you were a client, how would you want the home care aide collecting your specimens to act?

4.
What do you think are the most important points a home care aide should remember about collecting specimens?

REVIEW

**Key Terms – Test your understanding of each of these first.
Then use each one once to fill in the incomplete statements below.**

urine specimens

urine, feces, and sputum

disposable gloves

inside surfaces

fresh-fractional

midstream clean-catch

24-hour

stool

sputum

1. When collecting a _____ specimen, scoop the amount indicated with a wooden tongue blade and place it in the specimen container.

2. When a pair of urine specimens is taken 30 minutes apart, the second is the _____ urine.

3. Home care aides are not allowed to collect blood specimens but regularly collect specimens of _____.

4. When collecting a _____ urine specimen, you will pour collected urine into a special container using a funnel and may refrigerate or ice it to prevent bacteria growth.

5. _____ must be free of feces, toilet paper, and other material.

6. A _____ urine specimen requires cleaning the perineal area and taking urine from the middle of the urine stream.

7. _____ specimens are mucous expectorated from the bronchial tubes and lungs.

8. Touching the _____ of specimen containers and lids will contaminate the specimen.

9. Always wear _____ and use Universal Precautions and aseptic technique when collecting specimens.

Vital Signs and Weight

Vital signs are indicators of health.

Your vital signs (**temperature, pulse rate, respiratory rate,** and **blood pressure**—or **TPR** and **BP**) provide a profile of your health. Like fingerprints, each person's profile is a little different, but there are normal ranges within which most people fall. Vital signs that are above or below normal are often symptoms of a disorder.

Changes in vital signs mean changes in the body's functioning—for better or worse.

A healthy body at rest has vital signs that don't change very much. Clients are first measured to establish a *baseline measurement* and later to see if there are changes. If temperature is rising, pulse is falling, etc., the client's condition is changing, and it must be reported immediately. If the changes are great enough, they may reflect a life-threatening condition.

Weight can also be an important measurement of health.

Weight is **not** considered a vital sign but is considered an important part of each person's profile of health. Changes in weight are carefully watched since they can mean important changes in a client's condition.

Home care aides are responsible for measuring vital signs and weight.

How often you measure will differ by client and be indicated by the supervising nurse. All measurements must be accurate since they can directly affect the client's treatment. **Any time you are uncertain of information or feel you may have made a mistake, start over.** Always write results clearly and follow your agency's reporting policy.

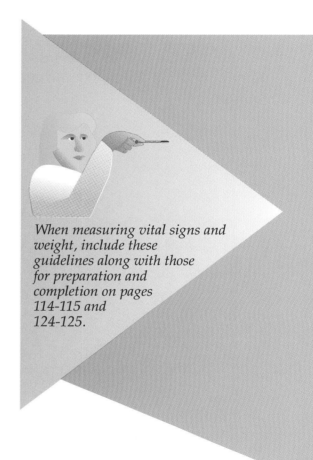

When measuring vital signs and weight, include these guidelines along with those for preparation and completion on pages 114-115 and 124-125.

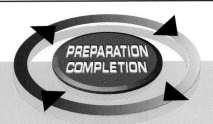

Communication

✔ Make sure you have a pen that works and paper on which to write results.

✔ Record results as soon as possible so you do not forget them.

✔ Record measurements correctly and according to agency policy.

Client Comfort

✔ The client should be at rest and in a comfortable position for the time it takes to measure.

✔ **Do not say anything or react in any way that will alarm the client** about results that may seem high, low, or changed.

Equipment

✔ Read and follow manufacturer's instructions for all electronic equipment. There are many varieties that do not all operate the same way.

✔ Handle glass thermometers carefully as they are breakable.

Safety

✔ **Be alert for abnormal readings or changes and report them immediately to your supervisor.** Remember that abnormal readings or major changes in vital signs may reflect a life-threatening condition.

✔ Clean all reusable equipment following agency policy and aseptic technique.

✔ When using electronic equipment, check electronic connections and outlets for safe conditions.

✔ **Follow aseptic practices and Universal Precautions when taking temperature.**

Temperature

The body produces heat and uses it to keep a warm environment for its systems.

This warmth is generally stable and is measured as a person's temperature. There are differences in normal temperature between people and within each person depending on age, activity, and other reasons. However, there is a normal range above or below which a client may be showing a symptom of a serious disorder.

You will regularly read clients' temperatures with a thermometer.

Fahrenheit is the temperature system used in the United States and *Centigrade* or *Celsius* is used in much of the rest of the world. Temperature is usually measured in the mouth *(Oral)*, but is also measured in the rectum *(Rectal)*, under the arms *(Axillary)*, and in the ears *(Tympanic)*. Glass thermometers require you to read the temperature. Electronic thermometers automatically read it for you.

Changes from normal temperature require immediate attention.

The normal range for oral temperature is 97.6-99.6 degrees Fahrenheit. *(On the Centigrade scale, this is 36.5°-37.5°.)* The normal range for rectal and tympanic temperature is 98.6°-99.6° Fahrenheit, and for axillary is 96.6-98.6°. **Readings above or below these ranges need to be reported to your supervisor immediately.** As temperature rises above 104 degrees, it can damage the body's systems and become life-threatening.

Temperature measurements must be accurate.

If you are not sure your reading is correct, take it again. Readings on glass thermometers should be quickly double-checked as it is easy to make a mistake in counting the cross-marks. Always record temperature readings as soon as possible so you won't forget them. Report clearly and correctly, following agency policy.

GLASS THERMOMETER

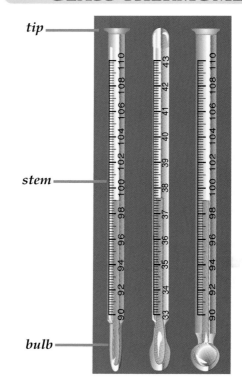

tip

stem

bulb

- The **oral thermometer** *(on the left)* has a long thin bulb of mercury and is often indicated with a *blue* tip.

- The **rectal** *(on the right)* has a thicker stem and a short round bulb to prevent injury to the rectum. It often has a *red* tip.

- The thermometer in the middle has features that allow it to be used for either oral or rectal readings. It is generally used with a plastic cover.

- Notice the difference in the Centigrade (middle) and Fahrenheit scales.

ASEPSIS AND PLASTIC COVERS

To reduce the risk of body fluid contamination, disposable plastic covers are used on all electronic probes and are widely used with glass thermometers (there are also disposable thermometers, though they are generally less accurate). **If you are using a glass thermometer without a plastic cover, you must disinfect and wash it before and after each use.**

ELECTRONIC THERMOMETER

TYMPANIC THERMOMETER

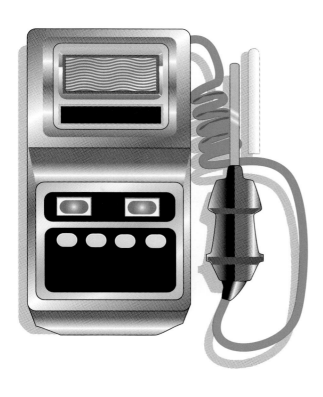

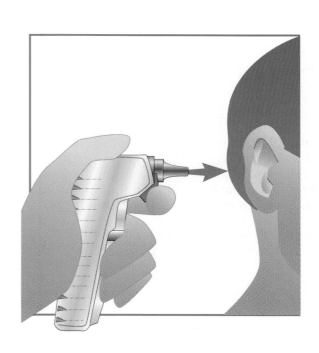

- Takes less time.
- Avoids mistakes by automatically recording temperature using a probe.
- Is battery operated, portable and easy to use.
- Is expensive by comparison to glass thermometers.

- Measures the temperature of the tympanic membrane and ear canal.
- Comes closest to measuring the body's internal ("core") temperature.
- Though generally the most expensive thermometer, is becoming more popular because of its speed and convenience.

Glass Thermometer

Body heat causes the mercury in a glass thermometer to expand along a line on which temperature is marked. Each long cross-mark is a full degree and each short cross-mark is two-tenths of a degree. The mark at which the mercury stops is the client's temperature. Though different types of thermometers are used for oral and rectal measurements, they must both be held in place for at least 3 minutes.

PROCEDURE

1. PREPARATION

- Follow the preparation guidelines on pages 114-115 as indicated by the Preparation Symbol. Pay special attention to the guidelines on *Vital Signs and Weight* on page 239.

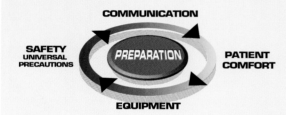

- **If you are using a glass thermometer without a plastic cover, disinfect and wash it before and after each use.** Wash with cold water. Never use hot.

- **Never use a thermometer that is chipped or cracked.** Check it first to see that it is not.

EQUIPMENT

- oral thermometer
- disposable plastic cover
- tissues
- pen and report form or paper

➡ *Glass thermometers will break if dropped or hit on a hard surface.*

➡ *Mercury is poisonous. Follow agency policy for reacting to leaked mercury from a broken thermometer.*

2. POSITION AND HOLD

- Hold the end of the stem firmly and shake the thermometer by snapping the wrist down. Repeat several times until mercury is clearly below markings.

- Put on disposable cover, if available. Ask the client to moisten lips. Insert and place the mercury bulb **under the tongue, slightly to the side.**

- Ask the client to close his or her lips over the thermometer and hold in place for **at least 3 minutes.**

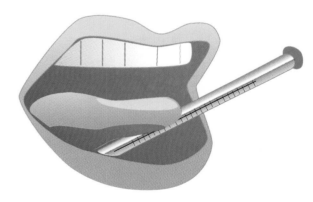

➡ *Oral temperature is not taken for at least fifteen minutes after a client has eaten, smoked, or had a cold or hot drink.*

➡ *Ask the client not to hold or bite the thermometer with his or her teeth.*

➡ *Axillary measurements require holding the thermometer in place in the center of the armpit for 9 minutes.*

POINTERS

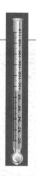

RECTAL MEASUREMENTS

Rectal readings are closer to the body's "core" temperature than oral. To take a rectal temperature, place the client in the Sims' position. Lubricate the rectal thermometer bulb (see page 240) and insert one inch into the rectum (one-half inch for infants). **Universal Precautions and aseptic technique must be used.** The thermometer is held for at least 3 minutes **while you support the client to prevent injury that could be caused if the client moves.** Use extreme caution since it is possible to puncture the rectum with the thermometer and cause severe injury.

3. REMOVE AND READ

- When ready, grasp stem and carefully remove as the client opens the mouth. Remove the plastic cover using tissues and dispose of both.

- Hold thermometer horizontally at **eye-level.** Turn it until the mercury becomes visible as a solid line.

- Note the temperature point at which the line of mercury stops by counting off the short cross-marks from the long. Double-check.

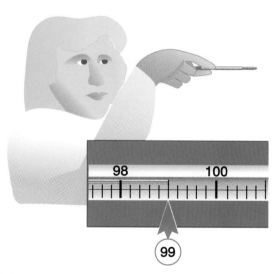

➡ *Never touch the bulb with your fingers while reading a temperature.*

➡ *Some thermometers have a long cross-mark to indicate 98.6 (the traditional number for body temperature). Don't confuse this with a full degree cross-mark.*

4. RECORD AND COMPLETE

- Record the temperature according to agency policy, followed by "O" for oral ("R" for rectal; "A" for axillary).

- Shake down thermometer. If you did not use a disposable plastic cover, disinfect and rinse the thermometer. Store according to agency guidelines.

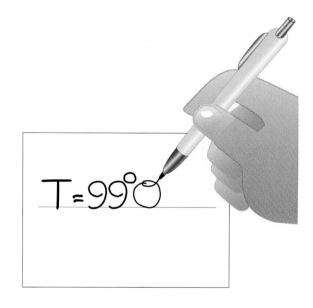

Follow the completion guidelines on pages 124-125 as indicated by the Completion Symbol. Pay special attention to the guidelines on *Vital Signs and Weight* on page 239.

Electronic Thermometers

An electronic thermometer uses a probe connected to a unit that automatically provides the temperature. You insert the probe into a cover and then place it in the mouth or rectum as you would a glass thermometer. The display on the unit flashes readings until it reaches the final temperature. It then generally sounds a tone and stops flashing. The unit is often hung from the neck using a carrying strap.

PROCEDURE

1. PREPARATION

- Follow the preparation guidelines on pages 114-115 as indicated by the Preparation Symbol. Pay special attention to the guidelines on *Vital Signs and Weight* on page 239.

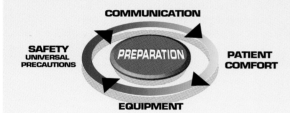

- Because of the many different types of electronic thermometers, be sure to follow the instructions for the unit you are using.

EQUIPMENT

- electronic thermometer
- correct probe or probe cover (red if rectal)
- manufacturer's instructions
- pen and report form or paper
- tissues
- (agency approved lubricant if taking rectal temperature.)

➡ *Electronic thermometers may allow you to choose fahrenheit or celsius (centigrade) readings.*

2. START UNIT

- Begin by hanging the unit around your neck with the display facing you.
- Remove probe from its receptacle to turn on the unit. (Some units will only turn on when a cover is installed.)
- Observe the start-up test. When ready, the unit will indicate "ON".

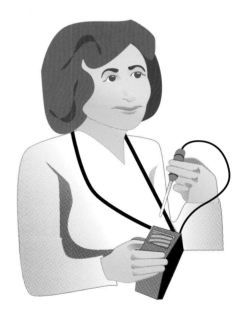

➡ *You may have to plug the probe into the unit if you are using it for the first time or if it has been stored unplugged.*

➡ **Be sure to use the correct probe for oral and rectal readings.**

POINTERS

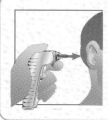

TYMPANIC THERMOMETERS

The probe of a tympanic thermometer is designed to fit in the client's ear. The unit is turned on by placing a cover on the probe. It is then positioned in the ear for one second. It measures the temperature of the tympanic membrane and ear canal. Because its measurement is closest to "core" temperature, rectal readings are unnecessary when a tympanic thermometer is available.

3. COVER PROBE AND POSITION

- Place a cover on the probe by inserting the probe into the probe cover holder. Grasp the probe carefully so you won't accidentally press the cover ejection button.

- Place the covered probe into the client's mouth as you would a glass thermometer. Position it according to manufacturer's directions.

4. HOLD AND RECORD

- Hold the thermometer in place yourself until the final temperature is reached. Remove and press the ejection button on the probe to dispose of the cover.

- Record the temperature according to agency policy, followed by "O" for oral or "R" for rectal. Replace probe in probe receptacle to clear the display and turn off the unit.

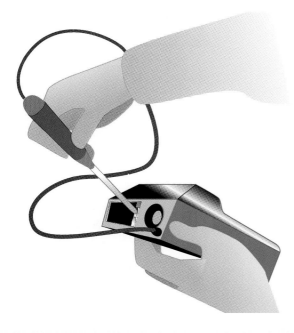

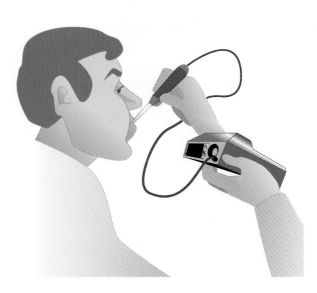

➡ *If taking a rectal reading, insert the probe a* **half inch** *into the rectum—note that this is different than with a glass thermometer. Lubricate the probe if necessary.*

Follow the completion guidelines on pages 124-125 as indicated by the Completion Symbol. Pay special attention to the guidelines on *Vital Signs and Weight* on page 239.

Pulse

Each heartbeat sends blood surging through the arteries, creating a pulse. The pulse is a measure of how often the heart beats and can be easily felt with your fingertips. Generally, you will check pulse at the wrist (radial artery), throat (carotid artery), and elbow (brachial artery). You will note the number of beats per minute and their regularity.

PROCEDURE

1. PREPARATION

- Review pages 60-61 on the *Cardiovascular System*, and note the major pulse points of the body.
- Follow the preparation guidelines on pages 114-115 as indicated by the Preparation Symbol. Pay special attention to the guidelines on *Vital Signs and Weight* on page 239.

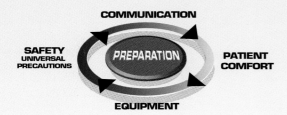

COMMUNICATION

SAFETY UNIVERSAL PRECAUTIONS

PREPARATION

PATIENT COMFORT

EQUIPMENT

- Position client for comfort either sitting or reclining.

EQUIPMENT

- watch that counts seconds
- pen and report form or paper

2. LOCATE THE PULSE

- Bare the client's wrist and place it palm-up, extended, resting on the bed or other surface.
- Feel for the pulse just above the client's wrist and thumb with the fingertips of your first three fingers.

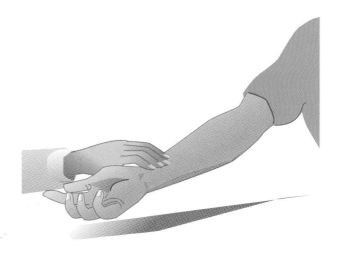

➡ *Make sure the client is completely relaxed, and has not just exercised or performed a demanding physical activity.*

➡ *If you cannot locate the radial pulse, try the brachial pulse inside the elbow.*

➡ *You cannot read a pulse with your thumb because the thumb has its own strong pulse.*

POINTERS

NORMAL PULSE

The normal range for adults is 60-100 beats per minute and slightly higher for children. Note that this can be affected upward or downward by exercise, stress, medication, illness, etc. A normal pulse should have a regular rhythm and force. Abnormalities in rate, rhythm and force should be reported to your supervisor immediately.

---

3. COUNT BEATS

- Look at your watch and choose a starting point you will find easy to read, remember, and use for calculation. Count the beats for 30 seconds and multiply by 2.

- Note if the pulse is irregular in rhythm or force. If so, count the pulse for a full minute.

4. RECORD AND COMPLETE

- Record the pulse rate according to agency policy. Notify your supervising nurse immediately if the pulse is abnormally low or high or changed from previous readings.

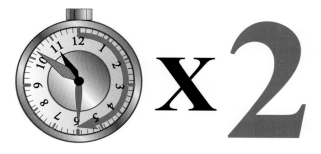

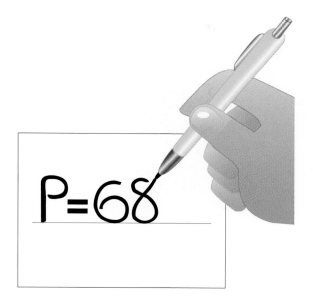

➡ *You may want to begin by counting for the full 60 seconds because it is easier to notice irregularities and you won't have to multiply the result.*

➡ *Be careful. It's easy to make a mistake reading or calculating seconds, especially since you are also counting beats.*

Follow the completion guidelines on pages 124-125 as indicated by the Completion Symbol. Pay special attention to the guidelines on *Vital Signs and Weight* on page 239.

Apical Pulse

The heartbeat is felt most strongly at the apical area of the heart, which is on the left side of the chest, a little below the left nipple. The apical pulse is taken by listening with a stethoscope for the sound of the heartbeat. Each heartbeat sounds as two quick sounds: "lub-dub." You listen for the number of beats per minute and their regularity, which you can observe by their sound.

PROCEDURE

1. PREPARE STETHOSCOPE

- Begin by following step 1 on page 246 for taking a pulse, adding a stethoscope and antiseptic wipes to your equipment.
- Wipe earpieces with antiseptic wipes. Place stethoscope earpieces in your ears.
- Warm the diaphragm against the palm of your hand.

2. POSITION AND LISTEN

- Uncover the apical area of the chest.
- Place the diaphragm of the stethoscope over the apical area directly against the client's skin.
- Count beats, record (indicating *Ap* after the rate), and complete following steps 3 and 4 on page 247 for taking a pulse.

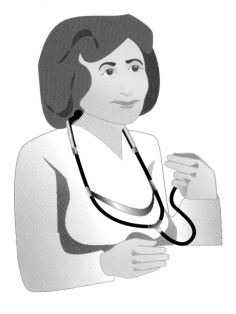

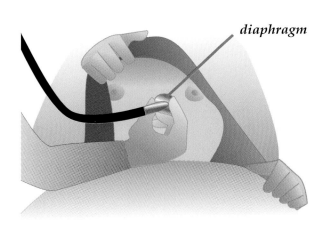

diaphragm

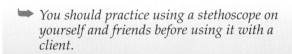 *You should practice using a stethoscope on yourself and friends before using it with a client.*

➡ *Listen carefully for irregularities in the loudness and type of sound.*

➡ *Be sure to maintain the client's privacy.*

POINTERS

Respiratory Rate

The *respiratory rate* is the number of breaths per minute a person takes. The normal range for adults is 14-20 breaths (or *respirations*) per minute. It is measured by watching the rise and fall of the chest. Each rise and fall is counted together as one respiration. Counting respirations is best performed with clients unaware of it so their breathing will be natural and unaffected. As a result, it is often taken with the pulse.

1. MAINTAIN PULSE POSITION

- Continue the position of feeling or listening for the pulse. Be sure to remember the pulse you have just taken.
- Watch for the chest to rise and note the time. Begin counting. Count each rise and fall as a single respiration.
- Observe the client for any signs of difficulty or pain.

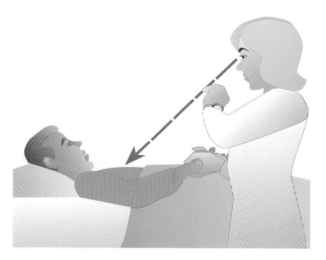

➡ *Respirations should be regularly spaced and quiet.*

➡ *You may want to begin by counting for the full 60 seconds because it is easier to notice irregularities and you won't have to multiply the result.*

2. COUNT AND OBSERVE

- Count for thirty seconds and multiply by two. If breathing is irregular in rhythm or sound, count for a full minute.
- Record pulse and respiratory rate according to agency policy. (You may be asked to record temperature, pulse, and respiration together: *TPR=99-68-18.*)
- Notify your supervising nurse immediately if either is abnormally low or high or changed from previous readings or if there are any irregularities.

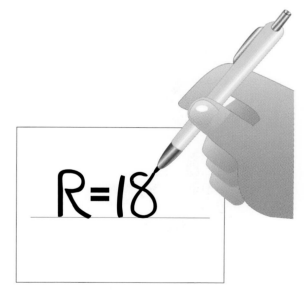

Follow the completion guidelines on pages 124-125 as indicated by the Completion Symbol. Pay special attention to the guidelines on *Vital Signs and Weight* on page 239.

Blood Pressure

Blood pressure is what forces blood through the arteries.

A *sphygmomanometer* (sfig-mo-ma-NOM-e-ter) is used to measure the outward pressure of the blood against the arteries. It measures it in two ways: *systolic* and *diastolic* pressure.

Systolic is the maximum pressure during heart contraction.

A systolic reading between 100 and 140 is considered normal in adults, though this will differ by client.

Diastolic is the minimum pressure when the heart relaxes.

A diastolic reading between 60 and 90 is considered normal in adults.

Blood pressure is written as a fraction with systolic over diastolic: e.g., 110/80.

Children have lower blood pressure and the elderly generally have higher. **Hypertension** is the condition of abnormally high pressure. **Hypotension** is abnormally low pressure.

There are different types of sphygmomanometers.

The most accurate use *mercury* (like a thermometer). An *aneroid sphygmomanometer* is one which measures pressure without a liquid. It uses a needle-type gauge that points to the pressure readings on a dial. There are also many types of *electronic* units which take automatic measurements. You must learn how to use the type available to you.

PROCEDURE

1. PREPARATION

- Follow the preparation guidelines on pages 114-115 as indicated by the Preparation Symbol. Pay special attention to the guidelines on *Vital Signs and Weight* on page 239.

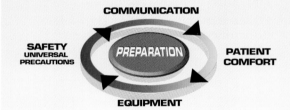

EQUIPMENT

- sphygmomanometer, with correct sized cuff
- stethoscope
- pen and report form or paper

➡ *Cuffs come in different sizes: regular, large, and pediatric. **Make sure you use the right size cuff,** one that fits easily around the arm.*

➡ *Make sure the client is completely relaxed, has not just exercised, and is not upset or feeling stressed.*

POINTERS

ABOUT THE PROCEDURE

- In measuring a client's blood pressure you will temporarily stop the circulation in the arm by inflating a cuff wrapped around the arm.

- When you deflate the cuff, blood flow will resume and you will be able to hear this through a stethoscope.

- A sensor in the cuff will indicate the amount of blood pressure in the brachial artery as circulation resumes.

- You will record the pressure indicated as you hear the sound described in the procedure below.

2. POSITION CLIENT

- Position client for comfort, either sitting or reclining. Position the arm on a pillow or surface so the arm is level with the client's heart.

- Bare the client's arm and place it palm-up, extended, resting on the bed or other surface.

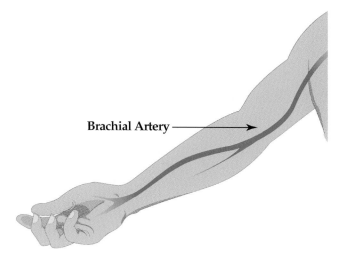

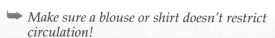

Brachial Artery

➡ *Make sure a blouse or shirt doesn't restrict circulation!*

➡ *Make sure the arm is straight.*

➡ *The brachial artery is found toward the inside of the arm*

3. PUT ON CUFF

- Check that the sphygmomanometer cuff is fully deflated.

- Wrap it snugly but not tightly around the arm approximately 1.5 inches above the elbow. Center the sensory device above the brachial artery.

- Position the gauge for easy reading.

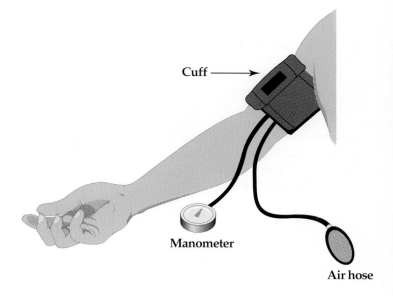

Cuff

Manometer

Air hose

➡ *Never put a cuff on an arm that has an injury or an IV.*

➡ *Many cuffs have an arrow or indicator for centering on the brachial artery.*

Blood Pressure (Cont'd)

4. CLOSE VALVE

- Place stethoscope earpieces in ears.
- Close the valve on the sphygmomanometer bulb.

5. INFLATE CUFF

- Locate the pulse on the brachial or radial artery (whichever is stronger) with your finger.
- Inflate the cuff 30 mm HG past the point at which you can no longer feel the pulse.
- Place the diaphragm of the stethoscope on the brachial artery above the inside of the elbow but below the cuff.

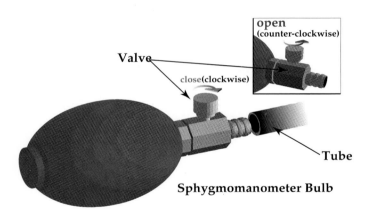

open
(counter-clockwise)

Valve

close(clockwise)

Tube

Sphygmomanometer Bulb

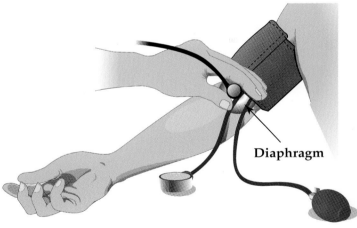

Diaphragm

➡ *For the first reading, a reasonable inflation range is between 170 and 200.*

➡ *If a client's blood pressure is consistent, you may stop inflating the cuff at any point at least 30mm HG above their usual systolic pressure.*

➡ *It's easier to locate the brachial pulse when the arm is straightened.*

ELECTRONIC BLOOD PRESSURE DEVICES

There are many Electronic Blood Pressure Devices available which measure blood pressure. These are especially popular for home use because they simplify the procedure by combining the functions of the stethoscope and the sphygmomanometer and by automatically measuring pressure. Specific directions for each device vary somewhat between models. Follow the directions for the model you use.

Note: readings taken on these devices need to be checked periodically against manually taken readings to make sure the device is accurate.

6. DEFLATE AND LISTEN

- Release the air in the cuff by opening the valve slowly. Note the gauge reading at the first pulse sound you hear on the stethoscope. **This is the systolic pressure.**
- Note the gauge reading when the pulse sound changes noticeably or disappears. **This is the diastolic pressure.**
- Remove stethoscope. Completely deflate and remove the cuff.

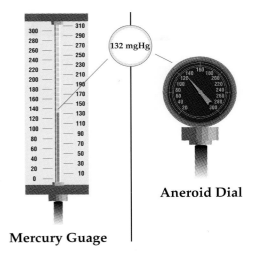

132 mgHg

Aneroid Dial

Mercury Guage

➥ *Turn the valve slowly and steadily so the cuff does not deflate too rapidly for you to get a reading. Be careful not to leave the cuff on too long or you will cut off circulation.*

➥ *The first time you take a reading you should measure the blood pressure in both arms. If pressure is unequal, measure the arm with the higher pressure thereafter.*

7. RECORD AND COMPLETE

- Record the systolic and diastolic readings according to agency policy. Indicate right or left arm and time of day.
- Follow the completion guidelines on pages 124-125 as indicated by the Completion Symbol. Pay special attention to the guidelines on *Vital Signs and Weight* on page 239.

Date	Time	Reading
10/22	8:00 a.m.	124/80 right arm
10/24	11:10 a.m.	132/80 right arm
10/26	8:00 a.m.	120/80 right arm

➥ *If for any reason you need to take another reading, you must completely deflate the cuff, pause to allow normal circulation to resume, and begin again.*

➥ *It's a good idea to practice taking measurements often and to have your instructor check your readings. You must be skilled at all steps of the procedure before working with clients.*

Weight

Weight can change with illnesses or certain conditions (such as edema or dehydration—see page 69). As a result, you may be asked to weigh some clients regularly. Most clients will have a common bathroom scale, but some may have the more precise balance scale. Steps 1-3 below are for using a balance scale. If you are using a common bath scale, see the notes at right.

PROCEDURE

1. CHECK SCALE

- Collect a paper towel and balance scale and follow the preparation guidelines on pages 114-115 and the guidelines on page 239.
- Help client remove footwear and unnecessary clothing. Place a paper towel on the scale.
- Check that the upper and lower weights are on zero and the balance arm is balanced with its pointer in the middle of the metal square.

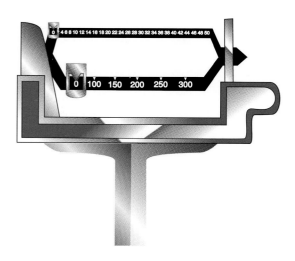

➡ *Be prepared to support the client if he or she starts to fall.*

➡ *Make sure the weights are resting exactly on zero. If the pointer still rests against the top or bottom of the square, the scale will need to be adjusted. Follow your agency's policy on this.*

2. POSITION LOWER WEIGHT

- Move the lower weight on the balance arm to the fifty pound mark that causes the arm to drop and the pointer to rest on the bottom of the metal square (A).
- Move it back to the previous mark so the pointer rises to the top of the square (B).

A
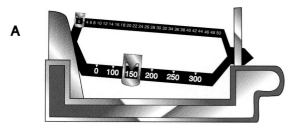

B
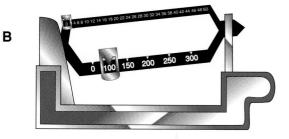

➡ *When the pointer rests against the bottom of the metal square, too much weight is set on the balance arm. Moving the bottom weight back one mark allows you to balance the arm with the right setting of the top weight in the next step.*

POINTERS

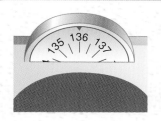

COMMON SCALES

If you do not have a balance scale, you can use a common bathroom scale which uses a dial to show weight. You should, however, check the scale's accuracy by weighing yourself on it and comparing this to your weight on a balance scale. Note the difference and report it to your supervisor.

3. BALANCE AND COMPLETE

- Move the upper weight to the pound mark that perfectly balances the pointer in the middle of the square.
- Add the lower and upper marks to get the client's weight. Record.
- Assist the client off the scale. Help him or her with clothing and footwear if necessary.

COMMON DIAL SCALE

- ✔ Make sure the client removes unnecessary clothing.
- ✔ Weigh the client at the same time of day.
- ✔ Make sure the dial of the scale is at zero before the client steps onto it.
- ✔ Make sure the client is steady and safe.
- ✔ Note weight when the dial stops moving.
- ✔ Help client off the scale.

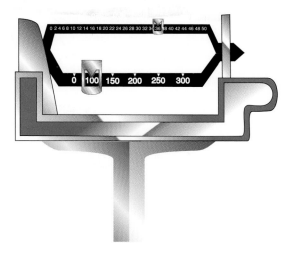

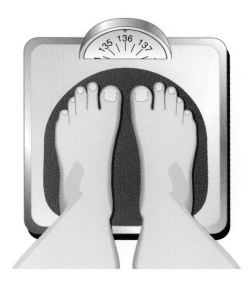

Follow the completion guidelines on pages 124-125 and the guidelines on *Vital Signs and Weight* on page 239.

➡ *Clients should use the same scale each time they are weighed so that differences can be noticed.*

Vital Signs and Weight

1.

What do you think the average client should know about temperature and blood pressure?

2.

Locate and feel your carotid, radial, and brachial pulses. What differences do you notice?

3.

Develop a profile of your vital signs by teaming with a classmate to take each other's. Compare your profile to the normal ranges for each vital sign. What does it tell you about yourself?

4.

What do you think are the most important points a home care aide should remember in measuring vital signs?

REVIEW

**Key Terms – Test your understanding of each of these first.
Then use each one once to fill in the incomplete statements below.**

TPR and BP

vital signs

temperature

oral and rectal

disposable plastic covers

tympanic thermometer

pulse

stethoscope

sphygmomanometer

systolic

diastolic

weight

1. The _____ is a measure of how often the heart beats and is felt by placing your fingertips against an artery.

2. When recording _____, "O, R, and A" stand for oral, rectal, and axillary.

3. Blood pressure is measured by using a _____.

4. The apical pulse is taken by listening with a _____ for the sound of the heartbeat.

5. _____ glass thermometers have different shapes.

6. _____ is not considered a vital sign but is an important part of each person's profile of health.

7. _____ are used on all electronic probes and are widely used with glass thermometers

8. _____ stand for an individual's vital signs: temperature, pulse rate, respiratory rate, and blood pressure.

9. The probe of a _____ is designed to fit in the client's ear.

10. If _____ are significantly above or below normal, they may indicate a life-threatening condition.

11. The peak blood pressure during heart contraction is _____ and the minimum pressure when the heart relaxes is _____.

Preventive and Restorative Care

Many clients require care that prevents certain disorders.

Decubitus ulcers (see pages 50-51), *muscle atrophy*, or *contractures* (see pages 54-55) are preventable disorders that are associated with bedrest and inactivity. Home care aides are responsible for providing basic skin care that keeps skin healthy and prevents the formation or spread of decubitus ulcers. They also assist in basic exercise therapy that prevents muscle atrophy or contractures and help clients with *medications* that maintain health or prevent disorders.

Restorative or *rehabilitative* care restores functions to the body systems after surgery or illness.

Non-sterile dressings are used to protect wounds and aid their recovery. *Range of motion exercises* restore muscle strength and flexibility to unused or injured muscles. *Deep-breathing exercises* help clients avoid respiratory disorders and rehabilitate impaired lungs. *Support bindings and stockings* control circulation and provide support to injured joints. Medications are also used as part of rehabilitative care.

The goal of preventive and restorative care is to maintain and restore as much function as possible in each client.

You will work with nurses, physicians, physical therapists, social workers, and others. *As a team,* you will provide care for the client's physical, psychological, social, and other needs. You will perform many of the activities described in this unit. However, your job description and agency policy will tell you specifically what care *you* are responsible for providing—and what you may *not* provide.

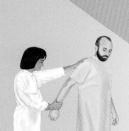

When providing preventive and restorative care, include these guidelines along with those for preparation and completion on pages 114-115 and 124-125.

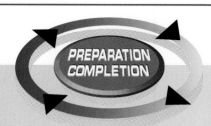

PREPARATION
COMPLETION

Client Comfort

✔ Report any client complaints of pain or discomfort directly to your supervisor. If you are providing care (such as range-of-motion exercises), stop immediately.

✔ Be especially sensitive to the client's feelings of helplessness, loss, or depression.

✔ Be especially sensitive to the client's privacy.

Communication

✔ Explain to the client the importance of telling you about discomfort or pain.

✔ Pay special attention to clients who cannot communicate easily: unconscious, cognitively impaired, infants, etc.

✔ **Always check the label before helping clients with medication and make sure you meet the *five rights of medication*.**

✔ Look for any changes in condition and report them immediately to your supervisor.

✔ Encourage the client to perform as much of an exercise as possible.

Equipment

✔ Follow manufacturer's instructions for pressure care devices and support stockings and bindings.

✔ Know which items are disposable and dispose of them after use.

Safety

✔ **Follow medication instructions exactly.**

✔ With range-of-motion exercises, **always support the joint. Move the joint as far as its free range-of-motion allows but never past the point of resistance or pain.**

✔ Observe the condition of a client's skin carefully, especially at the pressure points. Note any redness, blisters, or other signs of damage.

✔ **Never massage a reddened or inflamed area** as it will increase skin damage.

✔ **Use Universal Precautions when assisting with dressings.**

Decubitus Ulcers

Bedrest and inactivity can cause areas of the skin to break down.

Over time, pressure from the body's weight can block blood vessels at *pressure points*—places where the skeleton presses against muscle and skin tissue. If circulation is blocked long enough, the tissue dies and open skin sores called *decubitus ulcers* form. These ulcers are also called *bedsores* or *pressure sores* because they are associated with bedrest and pressure.

The skeleton's pressure points are the primary locations for decubitus ulcers.

The illustration at right shows the body's main pressure points. However, pressure from other causes (body parts, clothing, hard surfaces, etc.) can also lead to ulcers. In addition, skin damage from friction, moisture, or injury can help bedsores develop or make existing sores worse.

Prevention and early-warning identification are keys to keeping skin healthy and preventing decubitus ulcers.

Preventive care includes maintaining clean and dry skin, exercising regularly, frequent repositioning of inactive clients, and massage. Early symptoms of a decubitus problem are burning, tingling, or *inflammation* (redness, heat, swelling) which remain long after the pressure to the area is removed.

Home care aides provide care that prevents the formation or spread of decubitus ulcers.

Follow your agency's policies and the guidelines on these pages when providing skin care. Be alert for signs of problems and report them immediately to your supervisor. **Pay special attention to clients who are more likely to have decubitus problems:** clients who are frail, have poor nutrition, cannot move, are unconscious, or who are not aware of the need to turn.

PRESSURE POINTS

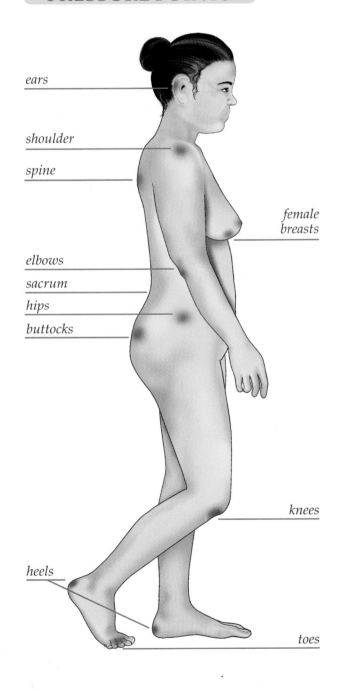

ears

shoulder

spine

female breasts

elbows

sacrum

hips

buttocks

knees

heels

toes

PREVENTION

When providing skin care, follow these guidelines and ask clients and their families to follow them when you are not there.

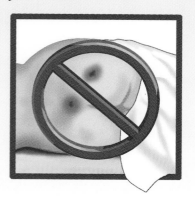

- Observe the client's skin carefully, especially at pressure points. Note any inflammation, blisters, or other signs of damage. Report them immediately to your supervisor.

- **Reposition clients frequently (at least every two hours),** avoiding movements that cause friction. For example, when repositioning clients in bed, lift or roll. Never drag.

- Assist the client to exercise regularly to increase circulation.

- Maintain clean and dry skin. Always pat the skin dry to avoid irritation.

- Make sure the bed is dry. Check incontinent clients frequently.

- Massage around affected areas but **never massage inflamed or irritated areas directly.**

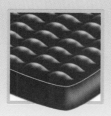

TREATMENT DEVICES

There are many devices that will relieve pressure on different parts of the body both to prevent the formation of decubitus ulcers and to heal them: cushions for different body parts, for the bed, for the wheelchair; electronic devices that automatically regulate pressure; and others. Always follow the manufacturer's and your supervisor's instructions when using these devices.

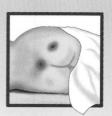

CLIENTS WITH DECUBITUS ULCERS

Only nurses and physicians may directly treat decubitus ulcers. However, you may provide skin care to areas *around* an ulcer and assist in ulcer treatment by repositioning clients, keeping clean and dry conditions, avoiding friction or pressure to affected areas, and by other methods ordered by your supervisor.

Non-sterile Dressings

Sterile technique prevents the introduction of any microorganisms to a wound. *Non-sterile technique* prevents the introduction of *harmful* microorganisms (pathogens) but not necessarily all microorganisms. Some wounds require a sterile technique in applying *dressings* (bandages). Some only need a clean or non-sterile technique. Home care aides often assist clients to apply *non-sterile dressings.*

To apply a non-sterile dressing, follow the steps on these pages.

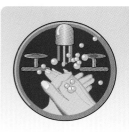

WASH HANDS.

Wash your hands before and after changing dressings. If there is any chance of drainage from the wound, put on **clean** disposable gloves.

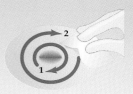

WASH "CLEAN" TO "DIRTY".

If cleaning the wound is ordered, clean wounds from the center of the wound outward. Wipe in full or half-circles, using a clean gauze pad for each wipe. Clean an area larger than the size of the dressing. Use your agency recommended cleaning solution.

DON'T OVER-TAPE.

Tape the dressing so it is secure but not "sealed" to the skin. That is, you generally should not cover the sides of a dressing with tape (unless ordered by your supervisor). Use only as much tape as necessary.

STERILIZATION

You can sterilize water (and any items you want to put in it) by boiling it in a covered pot for 10 minutes. You must allow time for the water to cool before using.

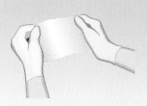

DON'T TOUCH.

The wound is considered clean. Do not touch the wound directly. The center of the new dressing must also be clean. Be careful not to touch any part of the dressing that will touch the wound.

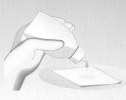

DON'T PULL.

If the dressing is stuck to the wound, soak it with sterile water. Then remove. Use baby oil or mineral oil to remove hard-to-loosen tape.

Follow preparation and completion guidelines on pages 114-115 and 124-125. Pay special attention to the guidelines on Preventive and Restorative Care on page 259. Collect all necessary equipment: tape, dressing, cleaning solution, gauze pads, trash bag, medication, etc.

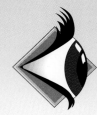

LOOK FOR CHANGES.

Observe the wound *and* the dressing. Look for swelling, redness, and drainage. Has drainage changed from clear to a yellowish-white pus? Is there blood in the drainage? Does it have a foul odor?

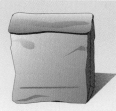

DISPOSE SAFELY.

If soiled dressings are contaminated by blood or body fluid, dispose in a plastic bag. If **not** contaminated by blood and body fluid, you may dispose in a paper bag. Note that your supervisor or the client's physician may want to see some soiled dressings themselves. In such cases, ask your supervisor for instructions.

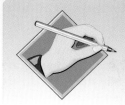

REPORT ACCURATELY.

Follow your agency policy. Note wound and dressing observations. Write clearly.

Medications

Physicians often order medications as part of the client's care.

These orders are called prescriptions. They must be filled by a pharmacist. A prescription includes the physician's instructions on how often and how much medicine to take.

Home care aides regularly assist clients with their medication.

Home care aides are generally not allowed to administer medications to clients. However, they often assist or remind clients to take their medication. They also **observe** the client's use or misuse of medication and are able to identify problems related to it. To do so, home care aides must be aware of each client's medication needs.

Prescription medications must be taken *as prescribed.*

Prescription medications may mean the difference between comfort and discomfort, illness and health, or even life and death. Failure to take them, taking them the wrong way, or taking the wrong amount can have serious consequences. If clients refuse to take medication, or if any other failure to follow the prescription occurs, you must report it to your supervisor immediately.

Many powerful medications are available without a prescription.

Decongestants, pain-relievers, and many other medications can be purchased *over-the-counter* at drug stores. While these may be safe in the doses recommended on their containers, excess usage or improper combination with other medications can cause problems. Home care aides should note any unusual consumption by clients of non-prescription medications and report it to their supervisor.

MEDICATION SAFETY

Medications taken improperly can be dangerous.

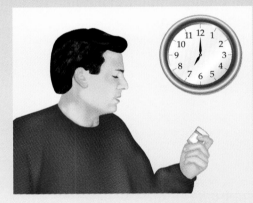

✔ Report all non-prescription drug usage to your supervisor.

✔ Be alert to clients taking multiple medications, especially from different physicians, and report it to your supervisor.

✔ Store as directed—always in a place safe from children.

✔ Never take prescription labels off containers.

✔ Always check the label before giving the medication to the client.

✔ Observe amounts of medicine in prescription containers to make sure client is taking doses correctly.

Some common abbreviations	b.i.d.	two times a day
that are used with	t.i.d	three times a day
prescription medications:	h.s.	bedtime
	q.o.d.	every other day
	p.o.	by mouth
	p.r.n.	as necessary

*Always check the prescription label before clients take their medication to make sure you meet the **five rights of medication**.*

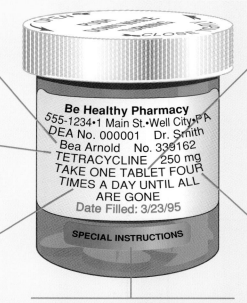

RIGHT CLIENT

The client's name must be the same as is indicated on the label.

RIGHT MEDICATION

The medication must be exactly as ordered on the care plan and as indicated to you in writing.

RIGHT DOSE

Make sure the client takes the amount indicated. Measure liquid amounts carefully.

Be Healthy Pharmacy
555-1234•1 Main St.•Well City,•PA
DEA No. 000001   Dr. Smith
Bea Arnold   No. 339162
TETRACYCLINE   250 mg
TAKE ONE TABLET FOUR
TIMES A DAY UNTIL ALL
ARE GONE
Date Filled: 3/23/95

SPECIAL INSTRUCTIONS

RIGHT ROUTE

A specific way to take the medication may be indicated: in the eye, on the skin, inhaled, etc. Oral medications (tablets, capsules, syrups, etc.) often do not have an indication. Check with your supervisor if there is any question.

RIGHT TIME

Doses are prescribed by the number of times in a day they should be taken, not the time of the day. This means you will have to know when the last dose was taken and when the next dose should be taken.

SPECIAL INSTRUCTIONS!

You must pay attention to any special instructions (*Take with food; Do not drink alcohol; etc.*) on a prescription container. They may be found on the label or on small stickers attached to the container.

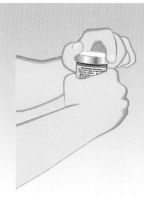

ASSISTING WITH MEDICATION

✔ Know before each visit what medication needs to be taken while you are there.

✔ Give the client advance notice of the time medication is due.

✔ Wash your hands before handling medication, glasses, or utensils.

✔ Check the label and make sure you meet the five rights.

✔ Open the container for the client if necessary.

✔ When the client is finished, store medicine and clean up as necessary.

✔ Note on the activity sheet or other form that the medication was taken.

✔ Make sure prescriptions are renewed *before* they are finished.

Exercise

Exercise is necessary to maintaining health and recovering from illness.

Exercise produces many health benefits, including stronger heart and lungs, lower cholesterol and blood pressure, increased joint and muscle flexibility, and improved balance and coordination.

Lack of exercise leads to serious physical problems.

Illness and aging often cause clients to be immobile for periods of time. As a result, muscles are not exercised and can waste away *(atrophy)* or tighten into deformed shapes *(contractures)*. This results in the loss of use of those muscles and a poorer quality of life.

The home care aide helps the client with exercise.

Exercises such as *ambulation* (walking) and *range of motion exercises* may be ordered as *therapy* for clients. They often require your assistance. Walking is one of the best forms of exercise but can be difficult and dangerous for the ill or elderly (See pages 182-183 on *Assisted Walking).* Range of motion exercises increase flexibility and strength in joints and muscles. They help clients keep or recover the normal range of motion needed for the activities of daily living.

All exercise can cause injury.

Walking can result in falling and range of motion exercises performed incorrectly can damage joints and muscles. You will be trained in proper exercise techniques and you must follow these and your agency's exercise guidelines carefully when assisting with client exercise.

Assisting client exercise is part of the home care aide's responsibility to help the client toward independence and a better quality of life.

therapy: The treatment of a disease or condition by medical or physical means other than surgery.

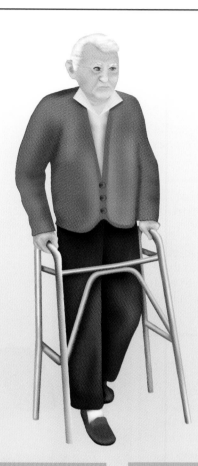

EXERCISE	LACK OF EXERCISE
✔ strengthens heart and lungs	✔ weakens many body systems
✔ improves circulation	✔ causes muscle atrophy
✔ lowers cholesterol and blood pressure	✔ causes muscle contracture
✔ increases joint and muscle flexibility	✔ leads to dependence and poorer quality of life
✔ strengthens muscles	
✔ improves balance and coordination	
✔ leads to independence and better quality of life	

Range-of-Motion Exercises

Muscles and joints must be used to keep their strength, flexibility, and function.

If a muscle is not active, it will decrease in size and strength *(atrophy)*. If it is not active for long enough, the muscle will deform into a *contracture* (see page 55) and stop functioning. Exercising joints and muscles with *range-of-motion (ROM) exercises* helps them keep or recover normal function.

Having normal muscle strength and joint range-of-motion is necessary for performing the activities of daily living.

Home care aides regularly provide range-of-motion care. ROM exercises are performed daily, often at the start of the day, and repeated later as needed with each client. They are usually performed with a client in bed, but can be done with a sitting or standing client.

Clients may perform range-of-motion exercises with or without assistance.

Always encourage the client to perform as much of the exercise as possible. *Active* exercise is performed completely by the client. *Passive* is performed by the home care aide. *Active-assisted* is performed partially by the client with the help of the home care aide.

Range-of-motion exercises performed improperly can cause injury.

They are always performed under the supervision of a nurse or physician. You must use extreme caution and a gentle technique. **Support the joint and never move past its free range-of-motion to a point of resistance or pain.** Stop at any signs of pain or discomfort and report them immediately to your supervisor.

Range-of-motion exercises are categorized by these types of movement.

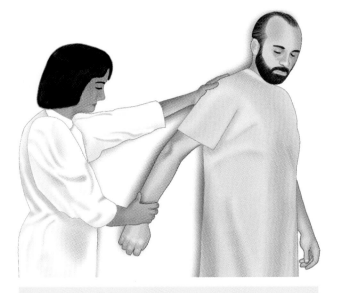

HYPEREXTENSION

Hyperextension is the *straightening past the normal position* to stretch the muscles and connective tissues of the joint. The client must be standing or sitting in a chair. When indicated, it must be performed with great care.

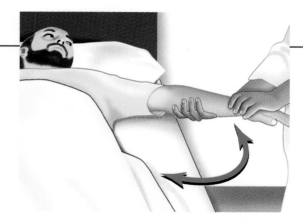

ABDUCTION/ADDUCTION

Abduction moves a body part away from the body or other body parts (as with fingers and toes).

Adduction is the opposite (*moves toward*).

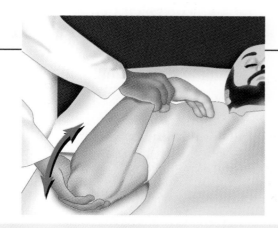

FLEXION/EXTENSION

Flexion is the *bending* of a limb or body part.

Extension is the opposite (*straightening*).

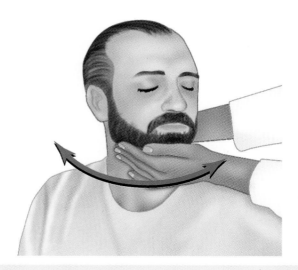

ROTATION

Rotation is the *circular turning of a joint.*

Internal rotation turns the joint *inward*, toward the center of the body.

External rotation turns the joint *outward*, away from the center of the body.

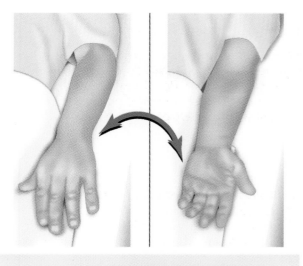

PRONATION/SUPINATION

Pronation is turning the joint down.

Supination is turning the joint up.

Range-of-Motion Exercises (cont'd)

PROCEDURE

1. PREPARATION & COMPLETION

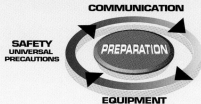

- To perform range-of-motion exercises, follow the preparation and completion guidelines on pages 114-115 and 124-125, and the guidelines on *Preventive and Restorative Care* on page 259.

- If using a hospital bed, position it at a comfortable height for you to work and lower the side rail on the side you are working. Exercise one side completely and then move to the other side. Use caution and a gentle technique. Keep body parts that are not being exercised covered. **Wash your hands.**

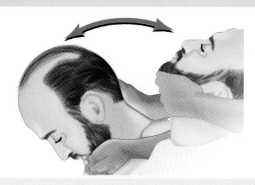

2. NECK

- Raise the client to Fowler's position. Remove pillow. Support the client's head by placing one hand under the chin and one behind the skull. Note: it is also acceptable to support the client's head with one hand on either side of the head, if that is more comfortable for the client.

- Tilt the head toward the chest (*flexion*). Straighten the head and neck (*extension*). Tilt the client's head back (*hyperextension*).

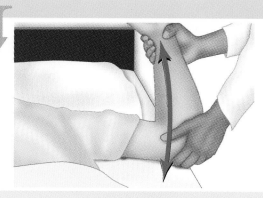

5. SHOULDER (cont'd)

- Bend the elbow 90 degrees and raise it level with the shoulder. Raise the forearm in an arc to rotate the shoulder (*external rotation*). Lower the forearm to the bed (*internal rotation*).

- Repeat each shoulder motion five times or as indicated.

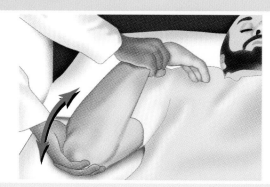

6. ELBOW

- Position the arm along the client's side and grasp it at the wrist and elbow. Raise the forearm in an arc so the fingers can touch the shoulder (*flexion*). Lower the arm so it is extends along the client's side (*extension*).

- Repeat each elbow motion five times or as indicated.

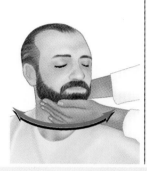
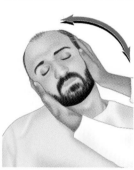

3. NECK (cont'd)

- Gently rotate the client's head in a circle *(rotation)*. Tilt the client's head from side to side *(lateral flexion)*.
- Repeat each neck joint motion five times or as indicated by the client's care plan. When finished, replace pillow and position client in the supine position.

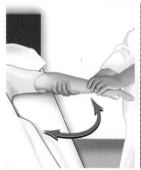
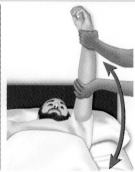

4. SHOULDER

- Grasp the client's arm at the wrist and elbow. Holding the arm straight, raise it in an arc over the client's head *(flexion)*. You may bend it to avoid hitting a headboard. Return it to his or her side *(extension)*.
- Move the arm outward from the client's side *(abduction)* and return it back *(adduction)*.

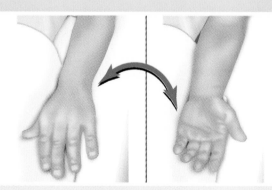

7. ELBOW (cont'd)

- Grasp the client's elbow and hand. Turn the hand palm-up to exercise the forearm *(supination)* and palm-down *(pronation)*.
- Repeat each forearm motion five times or as indicated.

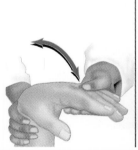
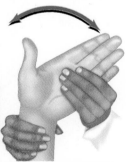

8. WRIST

- Grasp the wrist and palm. Bend the hand down *(flexion)*. Straighten *(extension)*. Then bend back *(hyperextension)*.
- Tilt the hand sideways toward the thumb side *(radial flexion)*. Then tilt it toward the little finger side *(ulnar flexion)*.
- Repeat each wrist motion five times or as indicated.

PROCEDURE

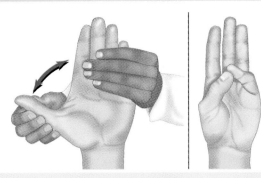 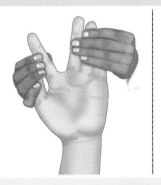 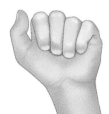

9. THUMB

- Grasp the thumb with one hand and the fingers with the other. Move the thumb toward the index finger *(adduction)*, then away *(abduction)*.
- Touch the thumb to each fingertip *(opposition)*. Bend the thumb into the palm *(flexion)*, then away *(extension)*.
- Repeat each thumb motion five times or as indicated.

10. FINGERS

- Grasp the fingers with both hands. Spread them apart one at a time *(abduction)*. Then bring them together *(adduction)*.
- Straighten the fingers *(extension)*. Then bend the fingers into the palm *(flexion)*.
- Repeat each finger motion five times or as indicated.

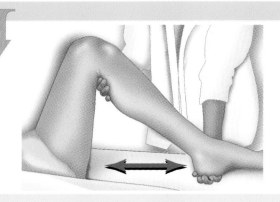 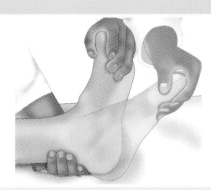

13. KNEE

- With one hand under the knee and one under the ankle, raise the knee and bend the lower leg back *(flexion)*. Then lower and straighten the leg *(extension)*.
- Repeat each knee motion five times or as indicated.

14. ANKLE

- Grasp the ankle with one hand and the foot with the other. Bend the foot up toward the leg *(dorsal flexion)*. Bend the foot down *(plantar flexion)*.
- Repeat each ankle motion five times or as indicated.

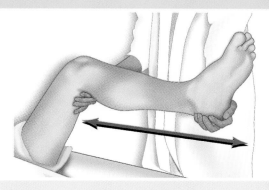

11. HIP

- Uncover the client's leg and place your hands under the knee and ankle. Bending the knee, raise the upper leg in an arc *(flexion)*. Lower and straighten the leg *(extension)*.
- Move the leg outward *(abduction)* and return it back *(adduction)*.

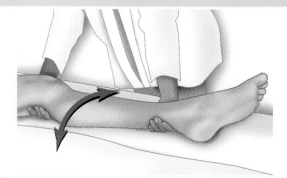

12. HIP (cont'd)

- Turn the leg inward *(internal rotation)*, then outward *(external rotation)*.
- Repeat each hip motion five times or as indicated.

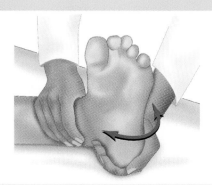

15. ANKLE (cont'd)

- Grasping the ankle with one hand and the foot with the other, turn the bottom of the foot toward the inside of the leg *(supination)*. Then turn it to the outside *(pronation)*.
- Repeat each foot motion five times or as indicated.

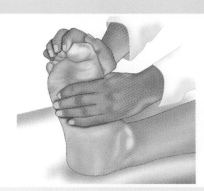

16. TOES

- Grasp the foot with one hand and the toes with the other. Bend the toes forward *(flexion)*, then back *(extension)*.
- Grasp the toes with both hands. Spread them apart one at a time *(abduction)*. Then bring them together *(adduction)*.
- Repeat each toes motion five times or as indicated.

COMPLETION

Assistive Devices

> **Assistive devices are devices which help a person to perform an activity.**

Many home care clients routinely use assistive devices to perform activities of daily living. Clients with limited hand control may use specially designed eating utensils, toothbrushes, hair brushes, etc. Many clients need glasses and hearing aids to see and hear properly. Others need walkers, canes, or wheelchairs to move about.

> **The use of assistive devices can contribute to the client's sense of self-esteem.**

Assistive devices allow the client to perform activities with less help from others. This increases the client's feelings of control, accomplishment, and independence, and in turn leads to better self-esteem.

> **Assistive devices are important tools in maintaining a client's ability to perform the activities of daily living.**

The health care team must routinely assess each client's need for assistive devices. As a home care aide, your observations about clients' need or use of assistive devices will be important in this assessment. You should always encourage clients in their use of assistive devices and report any problems you notice to your supervisor.

Assistive devices include:

DRESSING

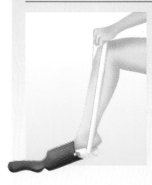

Among the devices which help clients to dress: sock and stocking aids which allow clients to pull on socks and stockings without bending; button and zipper aids which help clients with limited finger control to use buttons and zippers; and shoe-horns with long handles.

EATING UTENSILS

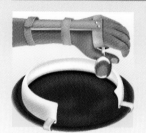

Many home care clients with physical disorders or disabilities use special eating utensils that allow them to feed themselves. Among the special utensils used are: forks, spoons, and cups with special handles; plate guards that help keep food on the plate; and special cutting tools.

PERSONAL CARE

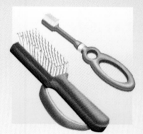

The ability to perform basic acts of hygiene and grooming is very important to self-esteem. Among the many assistive devices for personal care are: tooth brushes, hair brushes, and combs with special hand-grips; and bath brushes with long handles.

WHEELCHAIR AND TRANSFER

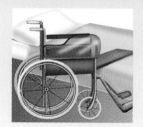

Wheelchairs are used by many clients, even those who are capable of walking but may be unsteady when they do. Armrests and other accessories are available to provide clients using wheelchairs with more comfort and convenience. *Transfer boards* are used to allow clients to move between the wheelchair and a bed or chair without assistance.

AMBULATION

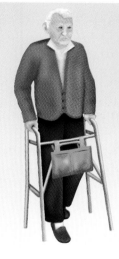

Walking is an excellent exercise for which many clients need assistance. There are many types of canes and walkers used to assist walking. Safety belts are also used. See *Assisted Walking* on pages 182-183.

Coughing and Deep-Breathing

Coughing and deep breathing exercises relieve lung congestion and help respiratory health. They are preventive care for clients for whom pneumonia or other respiratory disorders are a danger. They are restorative care for clients with respiratory disorders or who are recovering from surgery. How long and often they are done depends on the client and will be indicated by the supervising nurse.

PROCEDURE

1. PREPARATION

- Follow the preparation guidelines on pages 114-115 as indicated by the Preparation Symbol. Pay special attention to the guidelines on *Preventive and Restorative Care* on page 259.

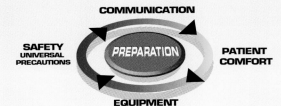

- Raise the client to a semi-Fowler's position. Fold back the covers from the rib and abdominal area.

EQUIPMENT

- disposable gloves
- small basin
- tissues
- pen and report form or paper

2. INHALE/EXHALE

- The client places his or her hands over the lower rib and abdominal area and then inhales deeply through the nose. He or she can feel the ribs and abdomen expand.

- The breath is held for a few seconds, and then exhaled slowly and completely. The ribs and abdomen should contract fully.

- Repeat 5 or more times as indicated.

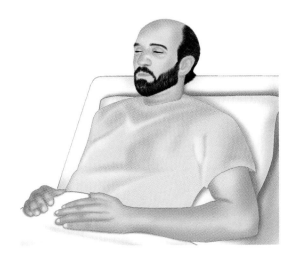

➥ *Coughing and deep-breathing exercises can be strenuous and painful. They are only performed under nursing supervision and will not be used with certain clients.*

➥ *Note and report any unusual sounds or signs of difficulty or pain.*

POINTERS

3. POSITION FOR COUGHING

- Because coughing is so strenuous, clients should support the abdomen with hand pressure (especially if there are any abdominal wounds). They can do so by locking hands over a pillow placed against the abdomen.
- **Put on gloves** in case any mucous is coughed up.

4. COUGH AND COMPLETE

- The client takes two or three deep breaths to prepare.
- Twice in a row, he or she inhales deeply, holds it briefly, and coughs out vigorously. The mouth should be kept open.
- Wipe any coughed-up mucous with tissues and dispose.

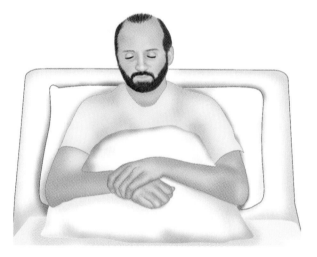

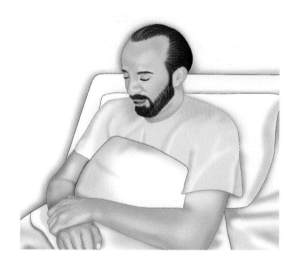

➡ *If you do not have an extra pillow, the client can press the palm of one hand against the abdomen and grasp that hand with the other.*

Follow the completion guidelines on pages 124-125 as indicated by the Completion Symbol. Pay special attention to the guidelines on *Preventive and Restorative Care* on page 259.

Stockings and Bindings

Stockings and bindings are used to provide support, prevent swelling, and assist circulation.

They apply pressure that supports weak or injured joints and are used to prevent swelling. *Anti-embolic stockings* are put on the legs to prevent the formation of blood clots caused by poor circulation. Some bindings use an electronic pump and compressed air to provide pressure.

Home care aides will apply anti-embolic stockings on some clients.

Blood clots (also called *thrombi*) form more easily when blood does not circulate freely. Once formed, clots can travel through the veins to other parts of the body where they can block blood flow. This blockage is called an *embolism.* The extra pressure of anti-embolic stockings assists circulation and helps prevent the formation of clots. They are generally put on at the start of the day before the client gets out of bed.

Stockings and bindings can restrict circulation and cause injury if incorrectly applied.

They are always applied under nursing supervision and must be checked regularly while being worn. They are removed at least twice during the day to allow normal circulation and are then reapplied. Some bindings are only applied by nurses. Learn and follow your agency's policy on stockings and bindings.

PROCEDURE

1. MEASURE SIZE

- Cover the client with a bath blanket. Fanfold down the top linens. Lift back the bath blanket to uncover the client's legs.

- Measure around the calf and thigh (the *circumference*) and the length of the leg to be covered. Use these measurements to get the correct size stocking as indicated by the manufacturer.

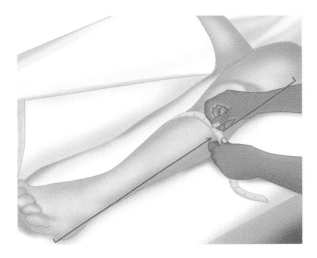

➡ *Observe the condition of the client's leg while you are measuring. Report any broken skin, infected areas, or other problems to your supervisor.*

➡ *If the legs are already swollen, your supervisor may ask you to elevate the client's legs for 20-30 minutes to reduce swelling.*

POINTERS

APPLYING ANTI-EMBOLIC STOCKINGS

To put on anti-embolic stockings, **begin by following the preparation guidelines on pages 114-115, the guidelines on** *Preventive and Restorative Care* **on page 259, and the stocking manufacturer's instructions.** Then, follow the steps below. You will need a bath blanket, tape measure, anti-embolic stockings, and manufacturer's instructions.

2. APPLY STOCKING

- Turn both stockings inside out down to the foot part of the stocking.
- Slip the opening over the client's toes and pull the stocking completely over the client's foot and heel.
- Bunch up the remaining stocking. Pull it up the leg, keeping it straight and smooth as you go. As the stocking is pulled over the leg, its seams should be on the outside.

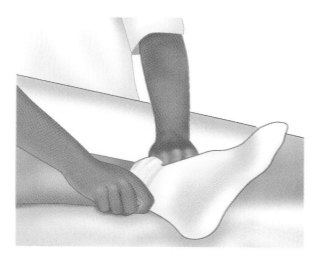

➡ *Always make sure the client's legs are level with the hips and not dangling when putting on stockings.*

➡ *Applying talcum powder to the legs will make putting on the stockings easier.*

3. COMPLETION

- Pull the stocking gradually and smoothly over the ankle and up the leg. Make sure it is on straight and there are no wrinkles. Repeat for the other leg.
- **Check the client regularly for discomfort or signs of swelling above the stocking.**
- **Stockings must be removed for at least a half-hour twice each day or as indicated by your supervisor.**

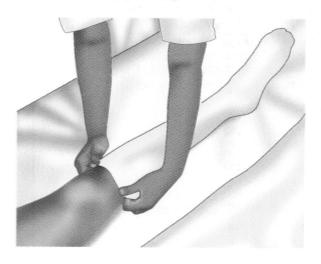

Follow the completion guidelines on pages 124-125 as indicated by the Completion Symbol. Pay special attention to the guidelines on *Preventive and Restorative Care* on page 259.

Preventive and Restorative Care

1.
What do you think the average client should know about bedrest and inactivity?

2.
What do you think are the most important points a home care aide should remember about medications?

3.
If you were a client receiving rehabilitative care, what would motivate you toward active self-care?

4.
What do you think the average client should know about range-of-motion exercises?

REVIEW

**Key Terms – Test your understanding of each of these first.
Then use each one once to fill in the incomplete statements below.**

preventable disorders

rehabilitation

pressure points

inflammation

five rights of medication

non-sterile dressings

range-of-motion (ROM)

active

coughing and deep-breathing

stockings and bindings

anti-embolic stockings

1. _____ exercises relieve lung congestion and help respiratory health.

2. _____ client exercise is performed completely by the client.

3. When assisting clients with their medication, always check the label and meet the _____.

4. _____ of the skin which remains long after pressure is removed is an early symptom of a decubitus problem.

5. The skeleton's _____ are the primary locations for decubitus ulcers.

6. _____ help prevent the formation of blood clots.

7. _____ is the process of restoring function to body systems.

8. _____ are used to provide support, prevent swelling, and assist circulation.

9. Decubitus ulcers, muscle atrophy, or contractures are _____ that are associated with bedrest and inactivity.

10. _____ exercises help joints and muscles maintain or recover normal functionality.

11. _____ require clean but not sterile technique.

POSTSCRIPT

We hope that this book has helped you build a good foundation for your career in health care. Successfully completing your training program and passing the competency evaluation is hard work. It is also a career accomplishment of which you can be proud. Now, you can advance your career by mastering your job as a home care aide and by continuing to learn all you can about health care and helping people.

Just as it was important to think about the information you were learning and to personalize it during your training program, it is important to do the same about your job as you perform it. Health care is a dynamic field. You will constantly be introduced to new situations, ideas, practices, and regulations that you must learn and master. Successfully doing so will bring you the appreciation of your clients and the health care professionals with whom you work. It will also bring you the satisfaction of a job well done. We wish you success.

Dennis Hogan

Publisher, Perspective Press

Glossary

abduction Exercising a body part by moving it away from the body or other body parts. 269

absorption The transfer of nutrients and water from the digestive system to the body's other systems. 67

active exercise Exercise performed by the client without assistance. 268

active-assisted exercise Exercise performed by the client with the assistance of another person. 268

activities of daily living The basic activities of health and hygiene that are required for independent living. 32, 274-275

adduction Exercising a body part by moving it toward the body or another body part. 269

AIDS Acquired Immune Deficiency Syndrome—a fatal disorder of the immune system. 63

Alzheimer's disease Disease with initial symptom of forgetfulness that progresses to total loss of emotional and intellectual control. 57

ambulation Walking. 174-175, 182-183, 266-267, 275

anatomy The structure of a body or organism. 49

androgens Male reproductive hormone. 59

anti-embolic stockings Stockings that apply pressure to the legs to assist circulation. 278

antibodies Chemicals that attack disease cells. 63

antigens Toxin (poison) or pathogen that causes an allergic reaction. 63

anus The opening at the bottom of the intestinal tract through which solid waste is eliminated. 67, 199

apical pulse Pulse measured at the heart using a stethoscope. 248

appendicular skeleton The skeleton of the arms legs and connecting bones. 52-53

appliance The disposable pouch which attaches over the stoma of an ostomy client for the collection of elimination. 224

arteriosclerosis Thickening and stiffening of the arterial walls. 61

arthritis A disorder that causes damage to the movable joints. 53

aseptic practice Maintaining clean, pathogen free or sterile conditions. 88

aspirating Breathing fluid into the lungs. 191

atrophy Shrinking and weakening of muscle from lack of use. 55

autonomic nervous system Nerves providing automatic regulation of body functions. 57

axial skeleton Skeleton covering the brain and spinal cord. 53

axillary temperature Temperature measured under the arms. 240

baseline measurement The first measurement of vital signs against which later measurements are compared. 238

bath thermometer A thermometer used to measure water temperature. 194, 200

battery Any unauthorized touching of another person. 21

bed bath A method for washing the client in bed. 194-197

bedpan A pan into which the client eliminates that can be positioned underneath the client in bed. 214

bedside commode A portable commode that can be wheeled to the client's room. 218

bedsores Areas where the skin and tissue underneath have died as a result of poor circulation caused by pressure. Also called decubitus ulcers or pressure sores. 51, 206, 260-261

bindings Used to provide support and prevent swelling. 278-279

biohazard The term used to indicate potentially infectious material. 91, 122

body mechanics Basic principles for lifting, moving, and positioning. 92-93

bowel movement The solid waste (feces) eliminated from the digestive tract, or the act of eliminating it. 212

brachial pulse Pulse measured at the brachial artery. 60, 246-247, 250-251

bursitis A joint disorder caused by repetitive motion. 53

capillaries The smallest blood vessels. 61

carbon dioxide The waste from the body's use of oxygen that is exhaled from the lungs. 65

cardiopulmonary resuscitation (CPR) The method of restarting the heart's pumping action for which special training is required. 104

cardiovascular Having to do with the heart, arteries, and veins. 61

care plan The home care team's plan for each client, with specific objectives and activities for that client's care. 26

carotid pulse Pulse measured at the carotid artery. 60, 105, 246-247

cartilage Connective tissue that holds the skeleton together. 53

catheter A device which uses a tube to drain urine directly from the client to a drainage bag. 220-221

Centigrade (also called Celsius) The temperature measurement system used through most of the world. 240

central nervous system The brain and spinal cord. 57

charting The recording of information in the client's record. 26-27

client's record The documents used to record each client's treatment and condition. 26-27, 28-29

clients' rights The basic rights to quality health care for every client established by federal law. 8

closed bed A bed that has been made with the top linens positioned to cover all or most of the bed. 151

cognitive impairment The inability of the brain to understand, remember, or think in normal ways. 34

colostomy The surgical creation of an opening to the colon. 225

commercial enemas Ready-to-apply enemas. 216

competency evaluation A written exam and a demonstration of skills required for employment as a home care aide. 19

condom catheter An external catheter that fits over the male penis. 222

confidentiality The requirement of the health care team to only record and discuss information essential to treatment and to keep all such information private among the health care team, the client, and the client's insurer. 9, 14-15, 28-29

constipation Irregular bowel movement or inability to have one. 67, 212

contracture Deforming and stiffening of muscle that causes loss of function. 55, 266

core temperature The body's internal temperature. 241, 245

cubic centimeters (cc) A fluid measurement. There are 30 cc's to an ounce. 142-143

cystitis Infection of the urinary system symptomized by frequent and painful urination. 69

dangling When the client sits on the edge of the bed with his or her legs hanging free. 170-171

decubitus ulcers Areas where the skin and tissue underneath have died as a result of poor circulation caused by pressure. Also called bedsores or pressure sores. 51, 206, 260-261

deep-breathing A breathing exercise to expand the lungs and promote respiratory health. 276

defecation The solid waste (feces) eliminated from the digestive tract, or the act of eliminating it. 212

dehydration The excessive output of water in the urine. 69

dementia Physiologically caused condition in which the ability to understand, remember, or think in normal ways is lost. 35

dentures False teeth that are form-fitted to the gums. 192-193

dermis The skin layer below the epidermis. 51

diabetes mellitus A disorder in which the pancreas does not produce enough insulin hormone to allow the body to use blood sugar. 59

diaphragm The respiratory muscle which most affects the expansion and contraction of the lungs. 65

diarrhea A condition where normally solid feces becomes liquid-like. 67

diastolic pressure The minimum blood pressure when the heart relaxes. 250

digestion The digestive system's breaking down of food and fluid into nutrients and water. 67

dorsal flexion Bending the foot up toward the leg. 273

drainage bag The bag attached to a catheter into which urine flows and is collected. 220, 223

draw sheet A short sheet positioned across the center of the mattress, often used for moving and positioning clients. 151, 162-163

dysphagia Difficulty in swallowing. 141

edema The excessive retention of fluid. 69

empathy Your ability to understand how other people see things. 24

endocrine system The system of glands which regulate the body the production of chemicals called hormones. 59

endometrium The lining of the uterus which collects blood in preparation for fertilization. 71

enema The injection of fluid into the rectum to create an urge to defecate. 216

epidermis The surface layer of skin. 51

epilepsy Condition of abnormal electrical activity in the brain resulting in convulsions. 57

estrogens Female reproductive hormone. 59

excretion The elimination of waste by the digestive system. 67

expectorate To cough up and spit out fluid. 235

extension Exercising a body part by straightening it. 269

external rotation Turning a joint outward. 269

Fahrenheit The temperature measurement system used in the United States. 240

false imprisonment Any unauthorized restraint of another person. 21

feces Solid waste from the digestive tract. Also called stool. 67, 212

finger sweep A method for removing food from the back of the mouth of a choking victim. 103

flexion Exercising a body part by bending it. 269

flow sheet A form for recording specific conditions or activities during brief periods of time. 27

fluid balance The amount of fluid the body must take in, put out, and maintain. 130-131, 142-143

fluid intake The amount of fluid taken in by clients through fluids and soft foods. 142-143

fluid output Generally measured as the amount of urine put out by the client (approximately 40% of total fluid output). 142-143

Fowler's position A sitting position for the client when the head of the bed is raised between 45 and 60 degrees. 159

fracture pan A smaller bedpan designed for clients with difficulty moving in bed. 215

fractures Broken bone. 53

fresh-fractional urine specimen Two urine specimens taken 30 minutes apart, the second being the fresh-fractional urine. 231

genitals The external sex organs. 69

graphic sheet A record of the client's vital signs that allows a visual comparison of results over a number of days. 27

Heimlich maneuver A method for forcing food out of the blocked airway of a choking victim. 100-103

hemorrhage Excessive bleeding from an external or internal wound. 107

hepatitis An infectious disease that attacks the liver. 67

HIV The virus which causes AIDS. 63

homeostasis The condition in which the metabolism stays at a level that allows the body to function best. 48

home care team All the people involved in the client's treatment: nursing, medical, service, and the client. 6-7

hospice A facility providing care for the dying and their families. 3

hygiene The degree of cleanliness and healthy conditions. 17, 186

hyperextension Straightening a body part past its normal position. 268

hypertension Abnormally high blood pressure. 261, 250

hypoallergenic tape Tape designed not to irritate the skin. 225

hypotension Abnormally low blood pressure. 250

hysterectomy The surgical removal of the uterus. 71

I&O record The written report of the client's intake and output. 27, 143

iliostomy The surgical creation of an opening to the small intestine. 225

immunity A barrier to disease created by the lymphatic system's production of antibodies. 63

incontinence The inability to control elimination, with unwanted leakage as a result. 212

indwelling catheter A tube inserted into the bladder to drain urine directly from it. 220

infertility The inability to reproduce. Also called sterility. 71

inflammation Redness, heat, or swelling of an area. 264

ingestion The taking of food and fluid into the digestive system. 67

intake and output (I&0) The foods and fluids taken in and feces and urine put out—of which fluid I&O is measured. 27, 134-135, 142-143

integumentary system The skin. 50-51

internal rotation Turning a joint inward. 269

intravenous tube (IV) A tube used to transfer nutrients, fluids, or medication directly into a vein. 141, 208

isolation precautions Safety practices which maintain a pathogen-proof barrier around a client to prevent the spread of contagious diseases. 90-91

job description The tasks and activities you will be expected to perform by your employer. 13

labia The lip-like opening to the vagina. 198

lateral flexion Bending a joint to the side. 271

lateral recumbent The position of the client lying on the side. 159

leg bag A catheter drainage bag that can be attached to the leg for client's who get out of bed. 222

lesions Open sores. 51

liability The legal responsibility you have for what you do that means you can be prosecuted for misconduct. 20

Licensed Practical Nurse (L.P.N.) A nurse who is licensed by the state but with less nursing education than the R.N. 7

ligaments Connective fibers that hold the skeleton together. 53

logrolling Turning the client while keeping the client's body completely straight and rigid. 168-169

Long-Term Care Facility (also called Nursing Homes) that provide basic day-to-day care and around-the-clock nursing service for the sick, disabled, or elderly who cannot provide it for themselves. 2-3

lymph nodes The organs of the lymphatic system which filter lymph for impurities. 63

lymph The fluid of the lymphatic system. 63

lymphoma Cancer of the lymph nodes. 63

meatus (urinary) The external opening to the urinary tract. 198-199, 220

mechanical lift A device to lift an immobile client out of bed using a sling and a hydraulic lift. 180-181

menopause The end of menstruation. 71

menstruation The shedding of the blood, endometrium and unfertilized egg if there has been no fertilization. 71

metabolism The physical and chemical processes by which the body's system functions. 48

midstream clean-catch specimen A specimen from the middle of the urine stream. 232

milliliter (ml) A fluid measurement. There are 30 milliliters to an ounce. 142

mitered corner A method of tucking in the ends and then the sides of bed linens at the mattress's corners. 149

minimum data set (MDS) A document for the complete assessment of the client completed by the interdisciplinary team. 26

multiple sclerosis Disease that gradually destroys the central nervous system. 57

negligence Failing to provide appropriate client care. 21

non-ambulatory A client who cannot walk. 178-179

nonverbal action How you physically communicate your attitude and other information without using words. 25

nutrients The elements of food (proteins, carbohydrates, vitamins, etc.) which the body uses for energy, maintenance, healing, and growth. 130

objective information Information you *see* as opposed to things you are told. 28, 125

occupied bed A bed with a client in it. 152-155

open bed A bed in which the top linens have been fan-folded back toward the foot of the bed to allow a client easier access to the bed. 151

oral hygiene Personal hygiene of the mouth, gums, and teeth or dentures. 190-191

oral temperature Temperature measured in the mouth. 240-243

osteoporosis A severe weakening of the bones. 53

ostomy belt A belt which attaches to the appliance to hold it in place. 225

ostomy The surgical creation of an opening through the abdomen to the digestive tract. 224

ova The egg of the female reproductive system. 71

paraplegia Paralysis of the legs. 57

Parkinson's disease Disease of the nervous system causing muscle tremors and spastic movement. 57

passive exercise Exercise of a client that is performed by the home care aide. 268

pathogens Viruses or microorganisms that cause disease. 88

penis The male organ for sexual intercourse. 71, 199

peripheral nervous system The nerves that carry information throughout the body and deliver it to the central nervous system. 57

personal dignity The quality of being worthy of respect and consideration—to which each client has a right. 8-9

personal hygiene Personal cleanliness and sanitary practice. 17, 186

personal toilet The process of personal cleaning or grooming. 196-197

physician's orders The physician's orders necessary for admission of a client. 26

physiological need The body's physical needs: eating, drinking, elimination, sexual contact, etc. 33

physiology The functions and processes of a body or organism. 49

plasma The liquid in the blood which carries the blood cells and platelets. 61

plastic draw sheet A short plastic sheet positioned across the center of the mattress to protect the mattress from fluid contamination. 149

pressure points Areas prone to decubitus ulcers where the skeleton presses against muscle and skin tissue. 260

pressure sores Areas where the skin and tissue underneath have died as a result of poor circulation caused by pressure. Also called bedsores or decubitus ulcers. 51, 206, 260-261

preventive care Care that prevents the development of a disease or disorder. 258

primary care The first care people receive, usually from a general practitioner who provides treatment for the day-to-day health problems that do not require specialized care. 2

privacy The right to keep all personal matters from general discussion, viewing, or knowledge—a right of every client. 8-9

pronation Turning a joint down. 269

prone The position of the client lying on his or her stomach. 159

prostate cancer Cancer of the male prostate organ. 71

pulmonary embolism The blockage of a lung artery by a blood clot. 65

pulse A measure of how often the heart beats. 246

pulse points The artery locations where the pulse is easiest to feel through the skin. 60

quadriplegia Paralysis of the arms and legs. 57

radial flexion Bending the hand toward the thumb side. 172

radial pulse Pulse measured at the radial artery. 92, 246-247

range-of-motion exercise (ROM) The exercise of joints and muscles to maintain or recover function. 268-273

rectal temperature Temperature measured in the rectum. 240, 243

Registered Nurse (R.N.) A licensed nurse with an advanced amount of nursing education who supervises the nursing team. 3, 6

rehabilitation Care that restores lost body function. 258

renal failure When the kidneys stop functioning. 69

respiratory rate The number of breaths (respirations) taken in a minute. 249

restorative care Care that restores lost body function. 258

rotation The circular turning of a joint. 269

safety belt A belt around the waist allowing others to lift or steady the client by grasping it. Also called a *transfer* or *gait belt*. 176-177, 182

secondary memory Recent or short-term memory. 57

seizures Uncontrollable temporary disorders characterized by fainting, loss of consciousness, and muscle spasms. 108

sensory information Information the body receives through the senses. 24-25, 51, 57

shampoo trough A basin designed for shampooing the client in bed. 202-203

Sims' position The position of the client in which the shoulders are nearly prone while the hips are in the lateral recumbent position. 159, 167

sitz bath A bath in which the client sits to soak the perineal area. 201

skin barrier A lotion, ointment, or (with ostomies) plastic barrier applied to the skin to protect it from irritation. 222, 224-225

sodium hypochlorite Household bleach that is diluted in water as a disinfectant. 123

specimen A sample that will be analyzed. 228

spermatozoa The male reproductive material necessary for fertilizing the female's egg. 71

sphygmomanometer A device for measuring blood pressure. 250

sputum Mucous from the lungs and bronchial tubes. 228, 235

sterile Microorganism-free conditions. 88

stethoscope A device for listening to internal body sounds such as the heartbeat. 248

stoma The opening to the digestive tract from an ostomy. 224

stool Solid waste from the digestive tract. Also called feces. 67

stool The solid waste (feces) eliminated from the digestive tract. 212

stroke An interruption of blood flow to the brain from a blockage or hemorrhage which damages or kills brain tissue. 109

subjective information Things you are told or guess at as opposed to things you see. 28, 123

sundowning A condition in which clients with dementia become confused or agitated late in the day. 35

supination Turning a joint up. 269

supine The position of the client lying on his or her back. 259

systolic pressure The peak blood pressure during heart contraction. 250

thrombi Blood clots. 278

24-hour urine specimen A collection of urine for a 24 hour period. 233

tympanic temperature Temperature measured in the ear. 240-243, 245

ulcers Areas where the intestinal lining has died. 67

ulnar flexion Bending the hand toward the little finger side. 272

Universal Precautions Safety practices for maintaining a protective barrier against blood-borne pathogens. 88-89

unoccupied bed An empty bed. 148-151

urinal A container designed for male urination. 219

urinary catheter A device which uses a tube to drain urine directly from the client to a drainage bag. 220-221

urinary meatus The external opening to the urinary tract. 198-199, 220

urine Liquid waste from the urinary system. Also called void. 69, 212

vaccine Substances that increase immunity. 63

venereal disease Any of a number of diseases contracted through sexual activity. 71

visitation The right of a client to visits by family and friends during reasonable hours. 8-9

vital signs A person's temperature, pulse, respiratory rate, and blood pressure. 238-239

void Liquid waste from the urinary system. Also called urine. 69, 212

walker A self-standing device that provides support for walking. 183, 275

INDEX

family, 7, 9, 36-37
fats, 130-131
feces, 67, 212
feeding a client, 140-141
femoral artery, 60
fertilization, 71
fiber, 130-131
fibrosis, 55
finger sweep, 103
fingernail care, 204-205
fire preparedness, 94-95
flatus, 67
flexion, 268-269
flossing (teeth), 190
flow sheet, 27
flu, 65
fluids, 130-131
food guide pyramid, 132-133
food stamps, 82
Fowler's position, 159
fracture pan, 215
fractures, 53
full liquid diet, 134

G

gait belt, 177
gall bladder, 66-67
gangrene 59
genitals, 71
general diet, 134-135
glands 58-59
gloves, 88, 120-121
gonads 58-59
gowns, 118-119
graphic sheet, 27
grooming, 186

H

hair follicle, 50-51
handwashing, 88-89, 116-117
health care team, 6-7
health, 16-17
heart attack, 61
heart, 60-61
Heimlich, maneuver, 100-102
hemorrhages, 107
hepatitis, 67
high-protein diet, 135
HIV virus, 63
home care agency, 2-3, 5-7
homeostasis, 48
honesty, 14-15
hormones, 59
hospice, 3
hospital bed, 147
housekeeping, 74-75, 76-77
hygiene 16-17, 186

hyperextension, 268-269
hypertension, 61, 250
hyperthyroidism, 59
hypotension, 250
hypothalamus, 56, 58-59
hypothyroidism, 57
hysterectomy, 71

I

iliostomy, 225
immune system (immunity), 62-63
in-service, 18-19
incident report, 89
incontinence, 69, 212
infants, 42
infection control, 88-89
infectious waste, 122-123
infertility, 71
inflammation (skin), 260
ingestion, 67
insulin, 59
intake and output (I&O), 27, 134-135, 142-143
integumentary system, 49-51
intravenous (IV) care, 141, 208
invasion of privacy, 20-21
involuntary (muscle action), 55
isolation precautions, 90-91

J

job description, 12-13
joints, 53

K

kidney disease, 69
kidneys, 68-69
kneading (massage), 207
Kübler-Ross, Elizabeth, 40

L

large intestine, 66-67
larynx, 64-65
lateral recumbent, 159
laundry, 78, 91
leg bag, 222
legal issues, 20-21
liability, 20-21
licensed practical nurse, (LPN) 7
lifting sheet, 162-163
ligaments, 53
linens, 149, 153
listening, 24-25
liver, 66-67
logrolling, 168-169
long-term care, 2-3
low-fat diet, 135
lung cancer, 65
lungs, 60-61, 64-65

FOUNDATIONS

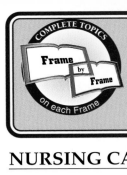

Index of Frames

Each pair of facing pages is a frame. It usually covers a complete topic. In a few cases, two topics are covered, and some procedures will take two or more frames. Use this handy index to quickly find the frame you want.

NURSING CARE